Veterinary Nursing Care Plans: Theory and Practice

Veterinary Nursing Care Plans: Theory and Practice

Helen Ballantyne PGDip BSc (Hons), RN, RVN

CRC Press
Taylor & Francis Group
Boca Raton London New York

CRC Press is an imprint of the
Taylor & Francis Group, an **informa** business

CRC Press
Taylor & Francis Group
6000 Broken Sound Parkway NW, Suite 300
Boca Raton, FL 33487-2742

Library of Congress Cataloging-in-Publication Data

Names: Ballantyne, Helen, author.
Title: Veterinary nursing care plans : theory and practice / Helen Ballantyne.
Description: Boca Raton : CRC Press, [2018] | Includes bibliographical references.
Identifiers: LCCN 2017034016| ISBN 9781498778664 (pbk. : alk. paper) | ISBN 9781138578104 (hardback : alk. paper) | ISBN 9781315155043 (Master eBook)
Subjects: LCSH: Veterinary nursing. | Nursing care plans. | MESH: Animal Diseases—nursing | Patient Care Planning | Veterinary Medicine—methods | Animal Technicians—education | Models, Nursing | United Kingdom
Classification: LCC SF774.5 .B35 2018 | NLM SF 774.5 | DDC 636.089/073—dc23
LC record available at https://lccn.loc.gov/2017034016
Typeset in Sabon LT Std Roman
by diacriTech, Chennai

Visit the Taylor & Francis Web site at
http://www.taylorandfrancis.com

and the CRC Press Web site at
http://www.crcpress.com

Contents

Foreword

The concept of nursing models of care and care plans was first introduced to veterinary nursing in 1998, where it was being taught on the first veterinary nursing degree course. The joint degree, delivered by the Royal Veterinary College, Middlesex University and College of Animal Welfare, benefitted from the expertise of nursing lecturers from Middlesex University as well as experienced veterinary nurse educators. The collaboration between the veterinary nursing lecturers and human centred nursing team helped to establish nursing models of care into the veterinary nursing curriculum and lead to the development, in 2007, of the first model of care specifically for veterinary patients.

As veterinary nursing develops as a profession, it is essential that we focus on our unique abilities in providing holistic care for our patients. Our role, ultimately, is to ensure our patients are returned to their owners, able to resume their normal routine. So, it is essential that we find out what the normal routine is for our patients when they are admitted.

The authors' background in, firstly, veterinary nursing and then human centred nursing, enables her to write this book from a unique perspective. The book provides an excellent resource for both student veterinary nurses and registered veterinary nurses, particularly if they are involved in training and education. The examples given provide insight into how care plans may be incorporated into everyday practice.

This book compliments and builds on those chapters already written in other veterinary nursing textbooks on the subject. The author uses veterinary examples to support the human centred literature and provides context to a number of new concepts introduced throughout the book.

Hilary Orpet
Andrea Jeffery

Preface

Veterinary nursing is evolving. There is a pressing need for veterinary nurses to learn, to share and to develop their role to the very best of their ability. Consideration of nursing theory, the models of nursing and the use of care plans is part of that development and it is hoped that this textbook supports that learning.

Being able to learn from human-centred nursing puts veterinary nursing in the unique position of being able to avoid 'reinventing the wheel'. Veterinary nursing must examine what has happened, what is happening and what is predicted to happen in human-centred nursing and learn from it.

The aim of this book is not to support one way of thinking or one model of care. The aim is to offer a broad overview of some of the emerging concepts of care planning that are discussed within the context of veterinary nursing. It is hoped that after reading this book, veterinary nurses may either borrow tools from its pages or design their own tools to support care planning for their own approach to patient care no matter which species of the animal kingdom they are caring for.

Extrapolating information from human-centred nursing and applying it to veterinary nursing presents a unique challenge in terms of language. To clarify, the term 'owner' has been used throughout the text in relation to veterinary patients to differentiate from 'carer or family' of human patients. Furthermore, veterinary 'practice' is used as the standard term to refer to a veterinary healthcare environment, simply to differentiate between this and a human hospital.

The content of care plan examples throughout this text are brief. The author makes no apology for this. In her opinion, care plans need to be useful and any care plan that requires the need for grammar and punctuation are the types of care plans that usually end up reserved for nursing education. While that is important, care plans in practice should stimulate thought and holistic assessment which usually may be done just as effectively with one word as with twelve. Sometimes applying theory from a textbook to clinical practice can be difficult. Throughout this text, the author has included specific 'In Practice' sections to try and facilitate this process.

For those veterinary nurses looking for further projects, a greater depth of understanding and a pathway to more advanced practice, explore the 'further reflections' section at the end of each chapter. Primarily these are a selection of concepts or ideas that may well stand further investigation by those willing to ask questions and think a little deeper.

Please note that all names used in examples in this book are fictitious and are for illustrative purposes only.

Acknowledgments

I would like to gratefully acknowledge Papworth Hospital NHS Foundation Trust and Mill House Veterinary Hospital for their kind permission to reproduce examples of nursing documentation within this textbook.

I would also like to thank Fiona Andrew, Sam Morgan and Sue Badger for kindly reading a number of chapters and proving themselves as highly effective 'critical friends'. Thanks also to Ailsa Marks who fanned the flame of a little idea a couple of years ago.

I owe a debt of gratitude to my family, friends and colleagues who have put up with endless references to 'the book' while I used all my evenings and weekends to read and write – I'm coming out to play now! Special thanks to the Hooligan, for being a real partner.

Finally, to the Ipswich railway station customer services team, I thank you, so very very much.

Author

Helen Ballantyne, after graduating with a degree in Pharmacology in 2002, qualified as a veterinary nurse in 2005. Combining her passions for veterinary nursing and travel, she began a 8-year stint as a locum nurse working nationally and internationally, developing experience in referral medicine and surgery, charity practice, emergency nursing and exotics. During this time, she spent five years on the British Veterinary Nursing Association (BVNA) council in a variety of roles, culminating in her being awarded honorary membership in 2016.

In 2013, she qualified as a human-centred nurse taking up a position at the United Kingdom's largest specialist cardiothoracic hospital, Papworth NHS Foundation Trust. After two years working in intensive care, she moved to the transplant team. Within this role, she supports the ongoing care of patients, pre and post-transplant. She is also a member of the National Organ Retrieval team, on call to facilitate the collection of organs from deceased donors.

Helen remains a Registered Veterinary Nurse and has developed a strong interest in the principles of One Health, supporting collaborative practice between the medical and veterinary professions. She regularly lectures and writes about ideas and ways of working that may be shared between the professions to support clinical and professional practice.

As she goes to work, her friends and family take great delight in asking her, 'Is it humans or animals today?'

What are nursing care plans?

Chapter 1

An introduction to nursing theory

By the end of this chapter you will be able to

1. Define care planning and nursing care plans.
2. List the advantages of planning care and using nursing care plans in relation to patient care and professionalism in veterinary nursing.
3. Define nursing models of care.
4. Discuss the differences between the traditional medical model of care and holistic care.
5. Consider the factors that have influenced the use of nursing care plans in veterinary practice.

It would be easy to dismiss veterinary nursing care plans as a recent fad or fashion. It would be easy to disregard the care plan written by an enthusiastic nursing student as little more than a useful educational tool. However, care plans are not new and rather than being reserved for education, a well-written care plan can have benefits for patients, for their owners, and for the veterinary team who care for them.

Care planning and the care plan

The terms care planning and care plan do not mean the same thing. **Care planning** is the process of recognising a patient's actual and potential problems and selecting interventions to assist in addressing those problems. This is what all nurses have been doing since nursing began, albeit implicitly. It is what many nurses do subconsciously when they meet and greet their patients. **Care plans** are the written record of that care planning process and can be used as a tool in a number of situations to facilitate the care of patients. Essentially, care planning is the thinking, the preparation, and the care plans are the resulting record of that action, or proposed action.

In 1860, when Florence Nightingale [1] was carving out the foundation of the nursing profession, she allocated a section in her book to 'petty management'. She went on to explain that 'all the results of good nursing, may be utterly negativised by one defect: petty management, or in other words, by not knowing how to manage that what you do when you are there, shall be done when you are not there'. Essentially, she was saying that good care may be compromised if there is no plan in place to continue that care once a nurse goes off duty. She goes on to explain that fresh air to the patient is just as important at Tuesday at 10 o'clock when the nurse must be absent, as it is at 10 o'clock on Monday when the nurse is with the patient. For today's nurse, the tasks have changed, but the principle remains. Nursing care requires careful planning to ensure continuity and quality of care.

The medical model of nursing

Researching the way nurses traditionally ran hospital wards reveals evidence that care was very much focused on the tasks that needed doing rather than on the patients and their needs.

In 1973, a research project called, 'A study into nursing care', was commissioned by the Department of Health and Social Security [2] and administered by the Royal College of Nursing. The main objective was to develop techniques of measuring the effectiveness of nursing care in general hospitals, and it consisted of twelve individual studies. As part of this project Sylvia Lelan conducted a study into nursing communication which revealed some interesting details on the way nursing care was planned and delivered at that time. She explained that there were generally two methods of planning the nursing work on the ward, and both involved making lists. One method assigned individual nurses to specific roles for that shift. For example, Nurse S would be responsible for bed-making, Nurse T was directed to carry out bed baths, and Nurse U was directed to administer medicines or four hourly observations. The second method of care planning used a notebook to list patients who had specific care needs in common. For example, a dressing book that listed Mrs F, Mr G and Mr O as in need of wound care on a particular day, or bath books that listed the patients in need of support with personal hygiene. It is clear that nurses were very much focused on tasks. This way of working is what is referred to as the medical model of nursing.

This is a model in which a person is always considered as a complex set of anatomical parts and physiological systems. Any symptoms that may be exhibited will be due to a disruption in that anatomy or physiology. The treatment of the patient is directed entirely by the disease with which they suffer and consequently, nursing under the medical model encourages nurses to carry out tasks solely on the instruction of the physician. The care was always centred on the disease or malfunction rather than on the patient. Just like the example of Florence Nightingale, this demonstrates that nursing care has always been planned, albeit in a different way.

With this brief reflection on a small part of nursing history, it would be easy to assume that nursing in the 1970s was bad and nursing today is good. This is not the case; such conclusions cannot and should not be made in such a simplistic manner. First, it is very difficult to compare the healthcare service of then with now, as resources, patient needs, and staff training are all significantly different. Second, to dismiss the care provided before current times as inferior is short-sighted. As an interesting example, in 1960 Isabel Menzies [3] published her seminal work discussing, amongst many things, the emotional impact of nursing. Within her work she defended the medical model of nursing. She maintained that breaking the work of a ward down into lists of tasks protected the staff from anxiety as personal relationships were not established with patients and decision making was avoided. This is certainly an interesting point of view in today's working environment, where mental health problems are experienced by many health-care professionals. The key point is that a comparison of nursing across the years is too complex an issue for the pages of this text. Any such discussion must be contextualised to take into account the significant changes in nursing specifically and the health service generally.

Defining nursing

During the 1950s and 1960s there was a new emphasis on developing the knowledge base of human-centred nursing. This led to the specific consideration and development of the role of the nurse, of models of nursing, and of care planning. Starting in the 1950s, Hildegard Peplau, a mental health nurse, started to promote professional standards in nursing and introduced the idea of advanced nursing practice. She proposed, amongst others, theories around the nurse-patient relationship and stressed the importance of the nurse's ability to understand their own behaviours in order to help others.

In 1955 Virginia Henderson [4] developed one of the most widely used definitions of nursing. It was a definition that was adopted by the International Council of Nurses in 1960 and is still widely used to identify the role of the nurse today. Her description of the 'unique function of the nurse' follows:

> To assist the individual, sick, or well in the performance of those activities contributing to health or its recovery (or to a peaceful death) that he would perform unaided if he had the necessary strength, will, or knowledge. In addition, she [the nurse] helps the patient to carry out the therapeutic plan as initiated by the physician' and 'she also, as a member of a team helps others as they in turn help her to plan and carry out the total programme whether it be for the improvement of health or recovery from illness or support in death. (p. 22)

In 1966 Virginia Henderson went on to publish her book, *The Nature of Nursing: A Definition and Its Implication for Practice, Research and Education*. In it, she introduced her philosophy of nursing, describing how people have biological, psychological, social, and spiritual components. It was a philosophy of that moved the profession away from simply carrying out tasks as instructed by the doctor. She envisioned the practice of nursing as independent from the practice of doctors, emphasising the unique role of the nurse. She supported empathy with patients and believed nurses really needed to get to know their patients to understand their needs. It was the foundation of caring for people as individuals, concentrating on their specific needs. It was the beginning of the development of holistic care. **Holistic care** may be defined as 'a system of comprehensive or total patient care that considers the physical, social, economic, spiritual and emotional needs of the patient, his or her response to illness, and the effect of the illness on the ability to meet self-care needs' [5].

In practice – Basic holistic care

In veterinary nursing, a holistic approach may be illustrated in a basic change from referring to 'the blocked bladder in kennel five' to the use of the pet's name and subsequent consideration of that animal as a whole.

So, the 'blocked bladder in kennel five' becomes Bam-Bam, the 4-year-old domestic short hair with urethral obstruction, who has a penchant for escaping from the kennel whenever possible and is owned by Mr Smith, who is deaf and needs more support with communication. Each of these aspects are relevant to a nurse approaching the patient and the owner.

As part of her work in 1973, Sylvia Lelan [2] supported the philosophy of holistic care, discussing the idea that planning and implementing individual care might provide nurses with increased professional satisfaction since their work would be less fragmented. She also raised the point that in working within the medical model, patients may have been receiving treatments they did not need.

The holistic care model is supported by more recent definitions of nursing, such as the one published by the Royal College of Nursing in 2014 [6], which states that nursing is

The use of clinical judgement in the provision of care to enable people to improve, maintain, or recover health, to cope with health problems and to achieve the best possible quality of life, whatever their disease or disability, until death.

Training the first veterinary nurses

In contrast to the human-centred nurses who were developing theories and philosophies of nursing, veterinary nursing as a role with specific knowledge and training was only just starting. Throughout the 1950s, proposals to formalise the training for veterinary nurses in practice were being debated, with many being opposed to such a scheme. In listing the wide range of tasks that the new animal nurses might carry out, which included laboratory work, radiography, handling and restraint, and the sterilisation of instruments, one vet wrote to the Veterinary Record to register his opinion. He concluded his objection with, 'they will know so little about so much that they will be of very little use at all' [7]. Other concerns voiced were based on fears that trained animal nurses would replace younger, inexperienced graduate vets, robbing them of their employment.

In contrast, supporters of the scheme believed that having a trained animal nurse would provide valuable and much needed assistance to the veterinary surgeon, freeing them up from menial tasks such as preparation of surgical instruments and administration of medication. So, while human-centred nursing pioneers were putting the patient very firmly at the centre of nursing care, veterinary nursing was being considered very much as a task-based role, falling straight into the medical model.

While the first veterinary nurses (later changed to registered animal nursing auxiliaries [RANAs]) were qualifying from the RCVS training scheme in 1963, there was further work being done to move human-centred nursing away from the medical model of nursing. The nursing process was introduced in 1967 by Yura and Walsh [8] and placed on the UK nursing syllabus in 1977, and is still taught today. It consists of a cyclic process of assessment, planning, implementation, and evaluation. The nursing process was introduced to encourage nurses to use a more structured, systematic approach to their work. It promotes a clear problem-solving approach to nursing care, with a clear emphasis on planning the care of a patient.

It is a simple process that can be applied to veterinary nursing. In fact, it is probably applied almost without thinking each time an animal comes into the practice.

In practice – The nursing process

Mick is a 3-year-old dog who is booked in for an x-ray and needs an intravenous cannula for the administration of anaesthesia. This is a fairly routine task, one that most veterinary nurses will have performed many times. Almost automatically, most nurses will start **assessing** the patient, trying to establish whether Mick is friendly and likely to tolerate such an intervention. The nurse will consider where to try and obtain venous access, look at his leg to locate and palpate his vein. The procedure is then discussed and **planned** with the colleague who will be restraining Mick. Equipment is prepared so that it is easy to reach so the procedure can be **implemented** swiftly and easily. **Evaluation** of the procedure will be ongoing. The nurse retraining Mick will be observing and feeling whether he is anxious, aggressive or likely to try and escape. The nurse placing the cannula will take their time, make a new plan if they are not able to access the vein, perhaps use a different cannula, or ask a colleague to attempt it instead. Once placed, the line will be flushed, and evaluation continues as new interventions may be needed if Mick chews at his bandage or the line blocks.

Models of nursing

Models of nursing are representations of the way care is carried out. Walsh [9] describes the nursing process as a tool to provide structure to care delivery and models of nursing as tools to instruct on how care should be given. Models of care provide an emphasis of care or stimulate an attitude to nursing the patient, individual to the needs of that patient, whether it be with the goal of self-care or developing a relationship to educate owners on caring for patients. Recognisable models include Roper, Logan, and Tierney's activities of living model of nursing (1983), King's Theory of goal attainment (1971), and Orem's self-care deficit model (1971). More recently, and specific to veterinary nursing, there is the Orpet and Jeffery Ability Model (2007).

Models represent things, as a globe represents the world. Models of nursing are abstract and anecdotally many nurses struggle to place a nursing model definition into words and struggle even more to contextualise them to clinical practice. If it is accepted that models represent the way an action is carried out, incorporating the aims and the philosophy of the action, then this concept can be illustrated by applying it to an everyday activity such as food shopping. The process will be the same each week, a process of *assessing* what is needed, *planning* to go, the action of *going*, then beginning a process of *evaluation* of what might have been forgotten, or will run out before shopping again.

In the shopping example, the attitude and values that are applied to that task will vary from both person to person and from situation to situation, much like healthcare. So, a thrifty father of a large family, keen to try and save money and needing to keep to a strict budget, will approach the shopping slowly, thoughtfully, checking prices, remembering to take bags with him, and using money off vouchers. However, this is a time-consuming process and therefore requires time and energy to work within that budget.

Alternatively, a young, busy, professional woman might be in a hurry. She needs to get the job done quickly and cares little for budget, so she shops online; with a planned delivery, the job won't take as long. These are two very different approaches to the same task. Both people achieve the same thing, a well-stocked kitchen, but the way each person has gone about it varies depending on the background situation, the context, and the priorities at the time. The same applies for healthcare. The model of care, the attitudes, and emphasis of a nurse caring for a person who is chronically ill is likely to be different from that of an emergency involving an acutely ill person who demands life-saving care. Models of care are used alongside the nursing process and provide the detail that is required to enable nurses to plan and carry out appropriate care.

The benefits of planning nursing care

There are three main advantages in taking the time to plan nursing care. First, thinking through and planning the care of either animal or human can provide a clear opportunity to prepare the patient and the environment for the care interventions. Second, it enables the nurse and patient owner to set clear individualised goals for the treatment. Setting clear goals provides measurable targets so that treatment can be assessed and if necessary adjusted and changed. Finally, planning the care of a patient can stimulate a written care plan which may be used in a number of ways.

The benefits of planning nursing care

1. Comprehensive preparation can be facilitated.
2. Individualised, measurable treatment goals can be set.
3. A written record of the planning process can generate a care plan.

Advantages of using nursing care plans

Benefits for the patient
1. Facilitation of holistic care
2. Improved continuity of care

Professional benefits
1. Improved multidisciplinary teamworking
2. Stimulus for research and care measurement
3. Thorough documentation of patient care to support professional accountability
4. Valuable education tool
5. Increased revenue for veterinary practice
6. Improved public perception of the role of the veterinary nurse
7. Increased professional satisfaction for veterinary nurses

A thorough, individualised care plan is a useful document with several functions.

Primarily there are advantages for the patient. A care plan written using a relevant model of care will facilitate holistic care. The care plan can be used to support communication between colleagues, ensuring there is continuity of care. Continuity is defined as a consistent, unbroken or continued action. In the case of veterinary nursing, **continuity of care** is the consistent application of high quality, individualised nursing care. The differences in knowledge base and clinical experience between staff members may affect the quality of a patient's care. Nursing care plans take that into account and help to avoid differences in quality of care.

The secondary advantages of using nursing care plans are diverse and support the professional aspirations of veterinary nursing. They may improve teamworking and facilitate the involvement of different professionals on the same case through shared information (known as **multidisciplinary working**) to ensure that all the patients' needs are being met. A care plan might be a useful source of information for administrative staff, a referral specialist, or nursing manager. Care plans can be evaluated in retrospect and become a source of research information and a resource to measure the care that has been given. They can provide a written record of care to support professional accountability. The educational benefit of nursing care plans can stretch across levels of experience and expertise if used as stimulus for discussion and debate about specific cases. The use of nursing care plans for chronically ill patients being cared for by owners at home may raise awareness of the role and responsibilities of the VN and potentially increase practice revenue. Finally, the use of nursing care plans may empower veterinary nurses to work independently and advocate for their patients, potentially improving their levels of professional satisfaction.

The implicit use of care planning in veterinary nursing

The potential advantages of using nursing care plans are clear. However, if we look to the very essence of veterinary nursing, it may be speculated that in fact, veterinary nurses are more likely to be engaged with the planning process than their human-centred colleagues. Historically, veterinary nurses have worked under the remit of the medical model. However, the practicalities of the work have stimulated an implicit holistic approach of planning and individualised care.

Working with animals requires a specific set of skills; being able to plan ahead and prioritise the care given is an essential aspect of any intervention with animals. As a basic example, an animal cannot be asked to sit still with their fingers applying pressure to a venepuncture site while the nurse scrabbles around for a bandage. At that point, a Jack Russel terrier, a little irritated by the fact that a veterinary nurse has just stuck a needle in them, wants to be off, back into their kennel or back through the door that their owner was last seen disappearing through. Ensuring that all the necessary equipment is available saves time with human patients and helps with aseptic technique. However, breaking off in the middle of an intervention to fetch something will not lose a human-centred nurse the chance to perform that intervention altogether. Most human patients will forgive a short break in proceedings. While some animals will also welcome the distraction, not all will.

Another factor that may facilitate veterinary nurses being more adept at planning their care than human-centred nurses is resource management. Working within the public sector there is often little knowledge or acknowledgement of the cost of disposable items, for example, wound dressings and sterile supplies. There is usually a ready source of such resources with little impact on the nurse or patient should an expensive dressing be accidently opened and therefore need discarding. In contrast, in the privately-funded veterinary world, most vet nurses know and understand how much equipment costs. This may be because ordering is part of their role, or because they are responsible for charging the client for such materials. Veterinary nurses may have an investment in the business, either as financial partners or as managers, and therefore hold some responsibility for finances, which in turn contributes to profit and loss, and eventually, their wages. This may then have a direct impact on the planning they do before starting a case that requires expensive equipment. When a replacement either cannot be acquired quickly or is particularly expensive, it can be assumed there might be greater care and planning applied in using such equipment.

It could also be argued that when it comes to providing individualised care, VNs are already working with the individual needs of their patient in mind. VNs are generally used to dealing with different species and different conditions all in the same day. Consider the average ward of a veterinary hospital, with routine neutering cases, perhaps an orthopaedic patient, and a medical patient in for blood tests and imaging. This is in direct contrast to most hospital wards where patients are hospitalised in groups according to their similar symptoms, for example, the renal ward, cardiac care, and orthopaedic ward. So, while veterinary nursing doesn't have the luxury of a long history to reflect on and learn from, due to the nature of the work, veterinary nurses are already using the principles of individualised care that human-centred nurses have had to learn over the years.

So, if veterinary nurses are used to planning individualised care for their patient and their owners, why is it that documentation of that planning, in the form of nursing care plans, seems to be a recent trend? In the UK, veterinary nursing students have been learning about nursing care plans for several years; the subject has been included in the syllabus since 2006. The current education guidelines and syllabus outline that veterinary nurses should understand the principles of the nursing process and be able to apply them to care planning. They are taught how to contribute to care planning, follow a care plan, and review it as needed.

In the UK, veterinary nursing is moving through a period of transition, which is similar to the period experienced by human-centred nurses in the 1950s and 1960s. There is a movement towards ensuring that veterinary nursing care is holistic. The aim is to improve the quality of care and ensure that all the patients' needs are being met. It is possible that it is this period of change that has stimulated discussion and debate on the theory of veterinary nursing, the use of models of nursing and nursing care plans. This period of transition includes changes in the regulation of veterinary nursing. Since 2012, all newly-registered veterinary nurses make a declaration on the day they join the register, '*I PROMISE AND SOLEMNLY DECLARE that I will pursue the work of my profession with integrity and accept my responsibilities to the public, my clients, the profession and the Royal College of Veterinary Surgeons, and that, ABOVE ALL, my constant endeavor will be to ensure the health and welfare of animals committed to my care*' [10]. This declaration makes it clear that putting the patient at the centre of all care should be the very highest priority for veterinary nurses, stimulating the profession to look for tools to facilitate such practice. Potentially, a comprehensive nursing care plan may be a tool to stimulate patient-centred care and provide a record of the care given to support professional accountability.

In 2015, a new Royal College of Veterinary Surgeons (RCVS) Royal Charter came into effect which meant the regulation of veterinary nursing across the UK. Under the changes instructed in the charter, registered veterinary nurses must adhere to the RCVS Code of Professional Conduct for veterinary nurses and, in case of serious misconduct, be subject to the RCVS disciplinary system. The Code of Professional Conduct for Veterinary Nurses was put in place to protect public interest and to safeguard animal health and welfare. This has had a direct impact on veterinary nurses and the way they practice. It makes them personally accountable for their professional practice.

A further significant development is the evolution of veterinary nursing education. Veterinary nursing training has developed and become more standardised so that most veterinary nurses are now taught by highly qualified and experienced veterinary nurses, instead of veterinary surgeons. Theoretical education is supplemented with practical experience and reflective practice. Students are taught to think about what they see in practice and learn in the classroom. This stimulates debate, questioning and research. Furthermore, with more veterinary nurses qualifying through the degree route, being able to demonstrate an ability to research and investigate questions and problems is a key part of the programme. This may be another reason that nurses have sought out tools to support this work. A contemporary and comprehensive care plan can provide an excellent source of data for comparison, audit, and investigation.

There are also changes in our society that may be influencing the way veterinary nurses conduct themselves and their work. Patients are able to see the change in the UK National Health System (NHS) as it moves away from the very paternalistic medical model towards a holistic approach that supports patients in making decisions about their own healthcare. It is only natural that people may seek the same principles of care for their pets. Recent reports of poor nursing care within NHS hospitals and the resulting investigations have placed emphasis on quality of care and meeting the basic needs of patients. Anecdotally, the expectations of consumers are rising and the threat of litigation increases.

This combination of social, professional, and educational factors may all be contributing to a veterinary nursing profession keen to adapt their practice to the changing needs of their patients and their owners. Nursing care plans are probably the single most useful tool in addressing these factors.

Applying a definition of nursing to veterinary nursing

Despite all these factors playing a role in stimulating discussion and debate about nursing theory in the veterinary sector, there is one subject of discussion that is missing. While the definition of human-centred nursing has been debated for over fifty years, there is no clear, widely used definition of veterinary nursing and little to no evidence of any debate on the subject. Should such a debate start, it should be argued strongly that given the patient group and the specific way of working that is required for veterinary nursing, planning the care of animals must be part of any definition of the role.

Including care planning in a definition of veterinary nursing echoes the definition developed by Virginia Henderson in 1960 [4] for human-centred nursing. Furthermore, there are other recognisable aspects of her definition that vet nurses might identify with. Health promotion is a role that many veterinary nurses perform daily, through nurse consultations, tackling existing problems from obesity to puppy and kitten checks to promoting healthy living through regular vaccination, good nutrition and parasite control.

Working to help the recovery of animals from illness is also often part of the daily work of veterinary nursing. A peaceful death, as mentioned by Henderson, is perhaps an area of nursing that comes more easily to veterinary nurses than their human counterparts. From the beginning of veterinary practice, euthanasia is a part of working life and may also form part of a legitimate treatment plan. Veterinary nursing has therefore evolved with this as a central part of their role.

One significant problem with applying Henderson's definition to veterinary nursing is that it is missing a crucial aspect of the role of the veterinary nurse. The obvious difference between the animal patient and human patients is an ability to understand and process information and make decisions for themselves. Clearly animals are not able to do this and therefore must rely on their owners. Veterinary nursing, by virtue of its patient group, requires a carer-centred aspect, something not emphasised by Henderson. Looking to established human nursing theory, the most suitable example to draw on is from children's nursing. The 2003 World Health Organisation's definition [11] of children's nursing is clear, and includes 'recognition of the pivotal role of the family to the child's health and wellbeing' as a key role of the children's nurse. It goes on to emphasise the need for a partnership between the children's nurse and their family to provide care, promote health, and/or adjustment or adaptation to a chronic illness or long-term illness. It finishes by incorporating the need to ensure that adequate support and education is in place to facilitate family coping and understanding of healthcare responsibilities as necessary. Each of these factors, recognising and working with the patient's carers, establishing a partnership and facilitating understanding, and the ability to carry out care, are also aspects of a veterinary nurse's role. They are a key part of caregiving that must be planned and incorporated into any veterinary nursing care plan. Perhaps, somewhere in between the definition of a children's nurse and an adult nurse, there are the foundations of a definition of veterinary nursing just waiting to be extrapolated.

Review

- The use of nursing care plans represents a shift in the philosophy of veterinary nursing care of animals from a medical model to a holistic approach.
- Planning nursing care is not new. Due to the characteristics of their patients, veterinary nurses have always planned the care of their patients.
- Nursing care plans may benefit patient care and support the professional values of veterinary nurses.
- The nursing process provides a structured format of thinking to apply to problems and challenges.
- Nursing models are used within the nursing process to assess patients and enable care planning that accounts for all patient needs.

Further reflections

Veterinary nursing is undergoing significant changes, both practically and professionally, as clinical knowledge advances and professional accountability is implemented. Consider how much influence the need for professional accountability in veterinary nursing had on the development of nursing care plans. Do you think that nursing care plans would be used in practice if there had not been the significant changes in the professional status of the veterinary nurse? Is it possible to measure the impact of professional accountability on changes in nursing documentation? Can you think of any further changes in nursing documentation that might occur over the next five or ten years?

Access a copy of the BVNA/RCVS Veterinary Nursing Futures document and consider how nursing practice may continue to change.

References

1. Nightingale F (1969). *Notes on Nursing: What It Is and What It Is Not*. New York, NY: Dover Publications (original work published 1860).
2. Lelean S (1973). *Ready for Report Nurse?* London: Royal College of Nursing Publishing.
3. Menzies IEP (1960). A case study in the functioning of social systems as a defence against anxiety: A report on a study of the nursing service of a general hospital. *Human Relations*, 13, 95–121.
4. Henderson V (1960). *Basic Principles of Nursing Care*. London: ICN.
5. O'Toole (2013). *Mosby's Dictionary of Medicine, Nursing and Health Professions*. 9th ed. St. Louis, MO: Elsevier.
6. Royal College of Nursing (2014). *Defining Nursing*. London: Royal College of Nursing.
7. Johnson JE (26th February 1955). The scheme for animal nurses. *Veterinary Record*.
8. Yura H and Walsh M (1967). *The Nursing Process*. Norwalk, CT: Appleton-Century-Crofts.
9. Walsh M (2002). *Models and Critical Pathways in Clinical Nursing*. 2nd ed. Edinburgh: Bailliere Tindall.

10. Royal College of Veterinary Surgeons (2012). Declaration on Professional Registration [online]. Retrieved from http://www.rcvs.org.uk/advice-and-guidance/code-of-professional-conduct-for-veterinary-nurses/.
11. World Health Organisation (2003). *WHO Europe Children's Nursing Curriculum*. Geneva: World Health Organisation.

Further reading

Use the resources below to gain a wider perspective on the history, definition and theory of nursing.

1. *What Is Nursing? Exploring Theory and Practice*. Carol Hall and Dawn Ritchie (Learning Matters, 2009).
2. *Politics of Nursing*. Jane Salvage (Heinemann Nursing, 1985).
3. www.icn.ch – The International Council of Nursing.
4. *Nursing Care Plans Made Easy* (UK edition) – Emily Matthews (Wolters Kluwer Lippincott Williams and Wilkins, 2010).

Chapter 2

The veterinary nursing process

By the end of this chapter you will be able to

1. List the four stages of the nursing process.
2. Apply the principles of the nursing process to veterinary nursing.
3. Differentiate between subjective and objective data.
4. Recognise nursing diagnoses and appraise their application to veterinary nursing.
5. Explain how data obtained from an assessment may be used to create a nursing care plan.

The nursing process

The nursing process of assessment, planning, implementation, and evaluation was introduced by Yura and Walsh in 1967 to encourage nurses to use a more structured, systematic approach to their work. It was a significant step towards nurses addressing the individual needs of patients, rather than making assumptions about the care required based on a diagnosis or set of symptoms, which was the traditional medical model of nursing (Figure 2.1).

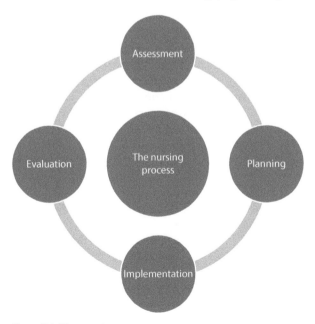

Figure 2.1 **The nursing process.**

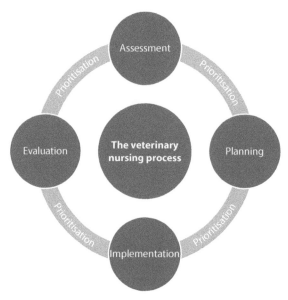

Figure 2.2 **The veterinary nursing process.**

Prioritisation

The nursing process can be used by veterinary nurses, with the addition of an extra step – prioritisation (Figure 2.2). The prioritisation of care, making sure the most important task is done first, is implicit within all nursing interventions and explicit in some assessment frameworks. Consider the very well-known ABC (airway, breathing, circulation) model in emergency first aid where checking an airway is prioritised over any other overt disease or injury. There is a clear instruction as to what to do and when. In veterinary nursing, prioritisation of care must be considered even before the assessment stage. When nursing people, information is usually gathered through a conversation and diagnostic tests, then a plan of care is made. The planned interventions can be prioritised according to a combination of clinical indication, patient decision, resource management, and timing. In veterinary nursing, the emphasis on prioritising care cannot be underestimated and needs to start before the assessment stage and weaved throughout the entire care process. The obvious difference between nursing people and animals is that people can be explained to and, if necessary, negotiated with. Animals do not offer that luxury. It is entirely possible that a veterinary nurse will have only one chance to assess their patient before they become too fractious to handle perhaps due to fear or pain. So, it is important for the nurse to decide in advance exactly what information they need to gather from the patient and how they will go about collecting that information.

Poor prioritisation of interventions can have a significant effect on the patient, the nurse, and potentially the day's work. Blundering into a kennel brandishing a stethoscope and thermometer without taking the time to learn a little about an animal can upset nervous or frightened patients.

Subsequently, data collected from an angry or agitated patient is unlikely to be reliable. The 'white coat syndrome' is well-established in human-centred nursing and manifests as a surge in blood pressure when it is measured within a clinical setting. It is an artificial hypertension as when measured at home, it returns to normal. This is also reflected in animals. With even the most laid-back animal, there may well still be some level of fear associated with being in the veterinary practice. It is a factor that needs to be taken into account when collecting data. Furthermore, an angry or agitated patient may also become a risk to their own safety and to the safety of the practice staff.

Additionally, as animals are often housed in wards with other patients, it is entirely possible that one fractious patient will spread fear amongst other patients who are able to perceive fear and stress. Finally, the impact of an agitated animal that is becoming too difficult to handle may be felt on a practice-wide level. The plan for the day may be disrupted by an unanticipated need for chemical restraint, altering the planned procedure significantly. Veterinary nurses need to understand the importance of taking the time to prioritise their assessment so they can gather as much information as possible before causing any stress or discomfort to the patient.

Prioritisation should continue throughout the care process. Each time the veterinary nurse approaches a patient, they should be asking themselves: what should I do first? What is the most important intervention? What can I do to ensure that I get the job done in the safest and most comfortable way for my patient? Keeping those questions in mind will facilitate a calm and measured approach to caring for animals.

Assessment

The assessment process consists of two sections:

1. Gathering information about the patient
2. Recording and communicating information

Gathering information

The aim of an assessment is to recognise actual health problems and potential health problems.

An assessment should be performed in a structured and measured way and nursing models support this part of the nursing process, facilitating a systematic approach. The information that may be collected as part of an assessment can be split into subjective data or objective data.

Both are equally important in the assessment process and both can be challenging to obtain.

Subjective data is generally qualitative, meaning descriptive information, and in human-centred nursing, is often defined simply as information that is obtained directly from the patient. However, nurses may also make subjective conclusions about their patients as part of their assessment; it is not always just information taken directly from the patient. It is any information that is based on opinion, emotion or interpretation. Experienced nurses, both human and animal centred, may observe certain behaviours and recognise patterns or responses in their patients that make suggestions and may influence their assessment conclusions. Such conclusions might be based on personal, or abstract concepts such as prior experience or intuition. The nurse may express, 'I have a feeling he is not right' or 'he looks like he is pain'. Both statements are subjective but relevant and, importantly, may prompt a nurse to carry out a full assessment revealing a previously undetected problem. Consideration of subjective data might be described as the 'art of nursing'.

In contrast, **objective data** is collected through the application of clinical skill, for example, counting a heart rate, observing respiratory rates, auscultating the chest, and measurement of parameters such as body temperature and blood pressure. Objective data is measurable and factual and is proposed as the 'science of nursing'.

Subjective data	Objective data
• Mood/demeanour	• Blood pressure measurements
• Itching	• Heart rate/breathing rate
• Pain	• Body temperature

Subjective data is usually gathered through obtaining a health history. Within human-centred nursing, this usually involves interviewing the patient, asking questions about their general health and well-being, before asking about the specific current problem. Clearly this is not an option open to veterinary nurses; the resource they rely on is the owner of the animal.

Understanding what is normal

One of the priorities of gathering a health history should be to establish what is normal for the patient. Learning patient routines including eating, drinking, and toileting patterns is essential to facilitate appropriate care. Offering the wrong food might lead to an erroneous diagnosis of inappetence. The author remembers caring for a dog belonging to an Italian family, who was superbly trained, but only to commands in Italian. This is a useful example of the need to understand the patient's 'normal'. Alongside establishing what might be considered normal husbandry for the animal, a normal health status should also be obtained. Information should be collected about any past medical history, whether the patient regularly takes medication and whether they have any ongoing health problems.

It is always worthwhile learning what is normal for the patient, even if it is not anticipated that an animal will stay in the practice overnight. Such information provides a baseline for that patient which subsequent observations might be compared to. It allows the veterinary nurse to replicate the patient's routine as much as possible with the aim of promoting patient comfort and, where possible, self-care.

Understanding the baseline of a patient's behaviour and routine can also contribute to being able to plan goals of care. Knowing what the animal was able to do before there was alteration in their health status allows realistic goals of care to be set. The concept of trying to understand what is normal for patients is applied throughout human-centred nursing, where most assessments are based on establishing what people are able to do unaided. The aim of such assessments is to promote patient independence and ongoing health. Within human centred nursing, there are specific tools used to ascertain baseline information before elective procedures. Patients are encouraged to complete detailed questionnaires to assist in care planning. Knowing in advance that a patient may live alone, or have several flights of stairs in their home may enable the team caring for them to put measures in place to faciliate a swift discharge from hospital with the necessary support to promote their recovery. Perhaps the same principles may be applied to veterinary patients? In both an elective and an emergency situation there may be appropriate times when an owner could be asked to complete details regarding their pet's normal routine, a valuable contribution to the care planning process.

After obtaining a health history the next stage is to perform a physical examination to obtain objective data. There are many methods of doing this, however, regardless of the framework selected, the principles are shared. There must be a methodical approach that ensures the animal is assessed holistically. A head to toe approach might be advocated, or a systems plan, gathering data on one body system at a time. It is recommended that a full assessment should be carried out each time an veterinary nurse begins to care for a patient. However, there is a caveat; assessments must be carried out within the context of the animal's condition. As an example, there would be little point in trotting an equine patient daily to assess for lameness, when they had been admitted for colic surgery.

The context of the assessment

Whilst gathering this information about the patient it is important to think about the context of the care required. An assessment requires the gathering of information both about actual problems and potential problems. The amount of information gathered will depend on the context of care.

So, in an emergency and acute care setting, after a dog has been hit by a car, there may be one specific health history question asked – do they have any medical conditions? – before moving on to the physical assessment to establish what injuries have been sustained and if any are actually life threatening or potentially life threatening. The health history is important, particularly if there have been diagnoses made in the past, however, it may not impact the current injury and so the questioning may be kept short and concise. Once the patient is stabilised, the health history may be resumed with the aim of trying to obtain a sense of what is normal for the patient in both their health status and their husbandry.

In comparison, an appointment to vaccinate a kitten will require a different approach. In this case the goal is health promotion. The emphasis of the assessment will be on subjective data. The assessor is trying to establish how the kitten is being cared for currently, gauging the owner's knowledge and understanding to establish if there is need for any improvements to the care being provided. Support materials in the form of written instructions might be offered and repeat appointments arranged. Both animals are being assessed but in very different ways, as one animal requires urgent care and the other requires long-term care through health promotion.

These different forms of an assessment are also reflected in human-centred nursing. A trauma nurse specialist attempting to triage multiple admissions uses a discrete assessment tool, rigid and concise, often with key trigger points to stimulate escalation of care where needed. However, a practice nurse, specialising in diabetes, is looking to promote self-management and therefore will begin a dialogue with the patient, asking for a self-assessment. They will try and establish how the patient is feeling, how they believe they are managing their diabetes, before addressing objective data and trying to establish how well the condition is being managed physiologically.

The use of assessment tools

The use of an assessment tool can be an extremely valuable adjuvant to the assessment process. Assessment tools contain a predefined set of triggers, usually a set of questions or indicators, to gather relevant and useful data. They facilitate the gathering of information that is known to help predict, screen or describe a condition or set of symptoms. The triggers can include subjective and objective data sets and usually lead to a clear conclusion regarding future treatment.

Assessment tools can be categorised by their function [1].

1. Health screening and diagnosis – These tools identify problems and usually assess their severity, e.g., a body condition score.
2. Descriptive – These tools facilitate the description of the problem in a clear and objective way, e.g., pain scores or stool chart.
3. Predictive – These tools facilitate the identification of potential problems through recognition of risk factors. In human-centred medicine, these are used frequently to anticipate and prevent hospital-acquired complications such as pressure area damage.

Consider the use of a pain score. After an invasive, soft tissue surgery, it can be assumed that an animal might be experiencing some level of discomfort. A pain score will take into account multiple indicators and may also generate a score based on how many indicators the animal is displaying that they are in pain. The more indicators they are displaying through their demeanour, body language or appetite, for example, the higher the score and the higher the likelihood the animal is in pain and the more likely there is need for additional pain relief.

There are several benefits to using assessment tools. Primarily, they will lend objectivity to potentially subjective data. This provides a way of considering health problems or potential health problems in terms that can be easily communicated to other professionals. Furthermore, completion of an assessment tool often leads to a clear numerical or staged conclusion. This is a valuable asset for comparison and evaluation once treatment courses have been implemented.

The other key advantage of using an assessment tool is the facility they have to support new or inexperienced staff. When a staff member needs to reach a conclusion about a particular patient's condition, it can be difficult to know exactly what to ask or what to look for to get the correct information. Assessment tools may minimise variation in assessment, which promotes continuity of care between staff members. Although, this does rely on the accurate and contemporaneous documentation of assessment tool results.

Benefits of using assessment tools

- Subjective data may be objectified to support continuity of care.
- Improved communication between team members occurs.
- They facilitate clear evaluation of care.
- They provide support for inexperienced members of staff.

Assessment tools in human-centred medicine

Within the NHS, assessment tools have a valuable role in resource management. If equipment is limited, assessment tools help healthcare professionals decide who should be provided with which equipment. As an example, all patients within the intensive care environment are regularly assessed for the likelihood of developing pressure area damage. Patients at high risk of developing areas of damage require preventative measures to be put in place, including the use of pressure-relieving equipment such as cushions or mattresses. However, this equipment is expensive and may be limited. Using an assessment tool enables the team to prioritise the equipment for the patients most at risk. Furthermore, the use of assessment tools provides evidence to support the procurement of further resources or equipment potentially facilitating change in practice and policy to support patient care.

A disadvantage to the use of assessment tools is the very technical terminology that is associated with them. This can be off-putting and exclude patients and their carers from discussions about their health status. Hearing their nutritional status described with a number, or their mobility with a falls risk level, may cause confusion and misunderstanding.

It is important that all team members using the assessment tool have a thorough knowledge and understanding of what the individual elements stand for and how they are used. Describing that a pain score has improved from three to zero will mean nothing unless there is some context and explanation. Both veterinary and medical staff must be able to interpret the conclusions and think about potential treatment plans.

Challenges to comprehensive assessment

Performing a holistic assessment within veterinary nursing may be challenging. Some animals are not going to allow nurses or vets to carry out a physical examination. In such cases, the emphasis will be on the health history provided by the owner. However, in situations of stress, owners of animals may not be able to remember parts of the patient's health history or may struggle to articulate the history clearly. It is the role of the veterinary nurse to encourage the admission of data. An animal's owner may have preconceived ideas as to the cause or even the diagnosis of a condition and it is essential that vets and nurses are not swayed by that and ask appropriate questions to gather all the relevant data.

The veterinary nurse will need to focus on detecting clues and signals from the patient that may indicate acute or chronic ill health. Being able to detect silent cues are an integral communication skill when working with people. Body language, behaviour, and attitude can all help direct a conversation. The same applies to animals. Observing a poorly kept coat, for example, doesn't require handling of the animal. However, it is a clue that the patient may have a chronic illness.

Poor record keeping can result in missed information from previous admissions or assessments which may lead to delays in diagnostics, omissions in care, and consequently, a compromise in patient safety. Information held on computer systems might also cause a barrier to information sharing as information might not be accessible to different care teams.

Communication and documentation of the assessment

A thorough assessment requires time and attention and a full assessment should always take place before any intervention is instigated (except in a life-threatening situation). However, the assessment process doesn't end once the information has been gathered. There is a need for clear and accurate documentation of the information gathered. Due to shift patterns or the need for particular clinical expertise, accurate documentation is required to facilitate the transfer of information between healthcare professionals. While information from a colleague can be extremely useful, nothing replaces gathering data independently. The author remembers looking after a patient in intensive care who was sedated and ventilated after undergoing a coronary artery bypass graft, and feeling slightly alarmed when reading that the previous nurse had documented that the patient's pupils were equal and reactive to light. This was certainly surprising as the patients left eye was in fact made of glass, so it would have been difficult induce it to react to light. It was clear that the previous nurse had not completed a neurological assessment and so held erroneous information about the health status of the person. Furthermore, it brought into question the other information that had been recorded during their shift.

Alongside comprehensive documentation, it is often beneficial to have a verbal exchange of information when transferring the care of a patient to a colleague. Communication frameworks are available to structure the presentation of verbal information. One commonly used tool used in human-centred healthcare was adapted from the U.S. navy, the SBAR tool [2]. This tool provides a template of communication to structure the transfer of information. The abbreviation stands for Situation, Background, Assessment and Recommendations. Originally developed for healthcare as a tool to support the escalation of care in acutely unwell patients, it is a model that might be applied easily by veterinary nurses in the same situation. Commonly, veterinary nurses are responsible for monitoring animals overnight, or in post-operative recovery. Using the SBAR tool facilitates the clear and concise transfer of information should the nurse have concerns about their patient and need to contact the duty vet. The situation is a short statement of the problem. The background provides brief information linked to the situation. The assessment should be a description of the objective and subjective data that has been obtained. The concluding recommendations are a description of the proposed action to address the concerns.

In practice – Using SBAR

Situation (short statement of the situation)

'I am concerned about Jess, I think that she has deteriorated'.

Background (information linked to the situation)

'Jess is the 7-year-old golden Labrador who was neutered this afternoon and extubated at 4 PM'.

Assessment (a report of the conclusions made after a full assessment)

'She was reluctant to go for a walk, so I checked her over. She has tachycardia with a rate of 140 beats per minute. She also has tachypnoea with a rate of 35. Her mucous membranes are pale, and her capillary refill time is greater than two seconds. She seems to be less responsive than she was earlier and her peripheral pulses are weaker too'.

Recommendation (a description of the proposed action)

'I would like you to come and assess her please. I think we may need to take some bloods, adjust her fluid therapy, and increase her analgesia'.

Planning care – Analysis of assessment information

The planning section of the nursing process is the stage where the information gathered in an assessment is analysed with a view to planning the care to be implemented.

Carpenito-Moyet [3] suggests three main areas of focus when analysing information collected in an assessment.

1. Strengths – The areas that the patient can draw upon to progress to previous or new health. In veterinary nursing terms, these are essentially the aspects of the patients' health that should not require any further intervention or assistance.
2. Risk factors – The things that might hold the patient back from recovery or progress, the potential problems.
3. Problems in functioning – The areas that are not functioning properly, the actual problems.

Nursing diagnosis

In analysing the data that has been collected through the assessment of the patient, a nursing diagnosis might be made. Forming a nursing diagnosis is advocated by many as an extra stage in the nursing process inserted between the assessment stage and planning stage. A nursing diagnosis is a specific label for each identified problem related to nursing care. The difference between a nursing diagnosis and a medical diagnosis is that the nursing diagnosis focuses on the overall care of the patient, taking into account all aspects of the patient's health and wellbeing, as opposed to just the physical symptoms.

In 1982 the North American Nursing Diagnosis Association (NANDA) was formed for the purpose of standardising nursing terminology. As part of their work, they created a list of over two hundred nursing diagnoses under 13 domains that range from physiological systems such as nutrition, elimination, and exchange to consideration of values, development, and growth. While some of these domains and the nursing diagnoses associated with them will not be relevant to animals, many are.

There are two significant points for the veterinary nursing profession. The first is the inclusion of the care of the family of the patient. Examples of nursing diagnosis related to family care include caregiver role strain and ineffective coping. Both are nursing diagnoses that, if missed, might influence the health of the veterinary patient in a negative way.

Second, the use of the NANDA standard diagnoses emphasises both actual and potential problems. For example, 'impaired skin integrity' and 'risk of impaired skin integrity,' are listed as formal nursing diagnoses. This emphasises the role of the nurse in preventative health by managing the risk factors that may slow a patient's recovery from illness.

Veterinary nurses may be anxious about using the term nursing diagnosis and it is seldom used in the UK. Veterinary nurses know and understand that the ability to diagnose medical problems is the basis of the delineation between the veterinary surgeon and the veterinary nurse. It is one of the fundamental differences between their roles. Given that the discussion of nursing care plans and holistic care is relatively new within veterinary nursing, it is understandable that there might be concern surrounding the use of nursing diagnosis. Using nursing diagnosis requires a comprehensive understanding of the roles and responsibilities of the nurse. It may be speculated that within veterinary nursing, where there is no universal professional definition, the role profile is not yet robust enough to facilitate front line staff confidence to differentiate clearly between nursing and medical diagnosis.

While the concerns around using the term diagnosis are acknowledged, many vet nurses will be using nursing diagnoses routinely, albeit implicitly. Consider a post-operative patient taking a long time to recover from their anaesthetic. The terminology that may be applied to the case, hypothermia, a common cause of prolonged recovery time, or risk of hypothermia, are NANDA nursing diagnoses. There are many terms used by nurses to describe the condition of their patients that are in fact NANDA nursing diagnoses. Therefore, instead of the nursing diagnosis being a separate stage of the nursing process, it might be considered part of the planning process, as a conclusion to the analysis of information gathered at the assessment stage.

The NANDA list of nursing diagnoses is worthy of consideration by the veterinary nursing community. It is a valuable tool reminding veterinary nurses of the wide range of care needs that should be assessed. There is also potential for further use of the concept of nursing diagnosis within veterinary nursing with the development of animal-specific nursing diagnoses.

Preparation for care

Once the information gathered at assessment has been assimilated and conclusions made, nursing interventions may be planned. One benefit of taking time to plan the care of a patient is that it allows care goals to be set. Care goals are a clear description of the aims and anticipated outcome associated with a nursing intervention. Such goals should address both actual and potential health problems. There is no point in placing a feeding tube in an animal that will not tolerate any handling. In this case, inappetence or an inability to eat is the actual problem and the animal's demeanour is a potential problem. Both problems must be taken into consideration when planning care or the care will not be effective.

While animals are hospitalised, often the veterinary nurse is the person who is monitoring their condition. Taking the time to set relevant care goals with the veterinary surgeon supports effective and efficient care. Parameters for vital signs can be set, then, should a reading fall outside the agreed parameters, pre-planned steps can be initiated and the veterinary nurse will feel confident in knowing when to seek assistance and escalate concerns.

Setting goals of care can also contribute towards improved continuity of care as all members of the healthcare team know and understand the priorities of care for the patient. In addition, explaining goals of care to the owners of patients can provide a deeper level of knowledge and understanding and may facilitate an improved compliance with the care required to try to meet the goals. Setting goals also provides a measure for the evaluation of the care given; an assessment may be made as to whether the goal has been met or not.

Spending time planning nursing care also allows the nurse to prepare the patient, themselves, and the environment for the care. This preparation can be either in the abstract, through thought and analysis, or through physical action.

Abstract preparation, thinking through the planned procedure, provides an opportunity to prioritise the nursing interventions. The veterinary nurse should always be thinking ahead, ensuring that they understand which tasks are the most important and should be carried out first. Equally important, the veterinary nurse needs to prepare themselves, asking whether they feel able to perform the procedure, checking that it is something within their scope of practice, and ensuring that their knowledge base is appropriate for the procedure.

Physical preparation is the gathering of the relevant equipment and assistance needed to carry out the care. Thorough physical preparation can be the difference between being able to perform an intervention or not. There is no advantage to preparing a patient for an x-ray if there is not the equipment to fulfil the plan. The animal is likely to become agitated if kept waiting. Poor preparation could also lead to extended sedation or anaesthetic times, potentially compromising patient health and safety.

Finally, the information gathered from the assessment and the associated planned care can be written down to form a nursing care plan. The care plan may include the goals of care as well as a list of interventions. Thinking the care through is care planning; writing down those thoughts makes a care plan.

Implementation of care

The third stage of the nursing process is the practical aspect of nursing; it is the stage where the planned care is carried out. Interventions are implemented to assist reaching the goals of care. There is no point in performing the most comprehensive assessment if the information is not going to be acted on. In fact, assessing the animal, noting problems, and then not acting on them could be argued to be a more serious deficit of care than performing a poor assessment in the first instance.

Evaluation

The final stage of the nursing process is simple. Evaluation is often perceived to be complicated and difficult to explain, but it is not. Everybody spends their entire day evaluating. Evaluating which route home will be the quickest during rush hour, evaluating which size packet of biscuits represents the best value for money, evaluating how much sleep is required and subsequently deciding what time to go to bed. Essentially, **evaluation** is checking that whatever is being done is having the anticipated outcome. Evaluating the care given to a patient is the method of checking to see whether it is improving the health of the patient as planned.

An evaluation needs to be comprehensive. Again, reflecting on how evaluation is carried out in general life, when evaluating whether a cake is cooked, takes more than a cursory glance through the oven window. The oven door should be opened, the cake needs to be looked at and possibly a skewer stuck into it to check it is cooked through. An evaluation of nursing care should be just as comprehensive. Primarily, the aim is to find out if the planned care goals been met. If the goal has not been reached, further assessment is required. Why were the goals not achieved? Why isn't the patient improving? Were the goals realistic? If the goals were met, does that signal the end of treatment? Or does it mean the next set of care goals may be set for the patient?

Do no harm

While it is important to ensure that the care given is assisting an unwell patient to recover, it is also important to check that after care, the patient is still able to perform the independent actions they were able to do beforehand. The whole patient must be assessed. After dressing an extensive wound, the bandage might well provide excellent healing support for a wound, however, if it impedes the animal from eating, there is an obvious need for adaptation and change. It is the process of evaluation that stimulates that adaptation and change. If the animal had not been checked after placement of the bandage it may have spent several hours without food and water.

The crucial point about the nursing process is that it is a cyclic way of thinking. The stages cannot and should not be performed in linear fashion starting with assessment and then ending with a single evaluation. Evaluation of care leads to further assessment and if necessary, the planning and prioritisation of new care goals, which will lead to further interventions and further evaluation, essentially beginning the nursing process cycle again. If a patient reacts badly to the use of noisy electric clippers, a nurse, acting out the nursing process, will not persevere with said clippers, chasing the animal around the practice, or pinning it down. They will reassess the situation and change their practice to achieve the care goal, and reach for the scissors.

This example illustrates how the nursing process is very often implicit in nursing actions and behaviours. Veterinary nurses are usually working with the nursing process in mind, sometimes without even knowing it. However, there are times when a more explicit use of the structure can benefit the process. Very often, this is when a veterinary nurse is presented with a situation they have not encountered before: an emergency, or a species, or set of symptoms that they are unfamiliar with. Here the nursing process may be invaluable in assisting the veterinary nurse to think carefully, plan their work and achieve the outcomes for the patient as they assess, plan, implement and evaluate.

Review

- The prioritisation of care should be a constant theme throughout the veterinary nursing process.
- Establishing what is normal for a patient helps support their comfort and care, and provides a valuable baseline with which to compare.
- Assessment tools have the potential to objectify potentially subjective data, making it easier to manage. However, they rely on all staff members having a thorough and robust understanding of their use.
- Planning care can facilitate thorough preparation for patient interventions.
- Evaluation of care is essential to ensure that the care provided is benefitting the patient.

Further reflections

The veterinary nursing process provides a structured way of addressing a problem or challenge. Try to apply that same process to your career, specifically your continuing professional development (CPD). The Royal College of Veterinary Surgeons advocates that veterinary nurses should take time to think about and plan their professional development so that their CPD is relevant to their practice and fulfils the criteria set by the Veterinary Nursing Code of Conduct.

Write down the stages of the veterinary nursing process and use them to structure your CPD plan. Reflect on your current knowledge level. What are your development priorities for the upcoming year? Are there any gaps in your knowledge you have recently identified? Is the practice purchasing a new piece of equipment that means you will need to learn new skills to use it?

Take the time to plan your CPD; think about when you will be able to do it. Are there any meetings or congresses you would like to attend? Document your plan and consult with your manager to establish whether you will have the support of your employer. Remember that CPD doesn't have to be expensive to be effective. Don't forget the benefits of learning from peers or working with the BVNA or the RCVS as council members. Finally, evaluate your plan throughout the year and update it as your priorities change or as opportunities for learning arise.

References

1. Barrett D, Wilson B, and Woollands A (2012). *Care Planning: A Guide for Nurses*. London: Taylor & Francis Group.
2. Institute of Healthcare Improvement (2017). SBAR: A Toolkit How to Guide [online]. Retrieved from http://www.ihi.org/resources/pages/tools/sbartoolkit.aspx.
3. Carpenito-Moyet L (2009). *Nursing Care Plans and Documentation*. London: Wolters Kluwer/Lippincott Williams & Wilkins.

Further reading

The following resources examine the stages of the nursing process in greater detail.

1. www.nanda.org – The Northern American Nursing Diagnosis Association.
2. *The Royal Marsden Hospital Manual of Clinical Nursing Procedures.* Lisa Dougherty and Sara Lister.
3. *Assessment Made Incredibly Easy* (UK edition). Helen Rushforth (Wolters Kluwer Lippincott Williams and Wilkins, 2010).
4. *Patient Assessment and Care Planning in Nursing.* Lioba Howatson-Jones, Mooi Standing and Susan Roberts (Learning Matters SAGE, 2015).

Chapter 3

Models of nursing care

By the end of this chapter you will be able to

1. State the functions of nursing models.
2. Identify the principles of the Roper, Logan and Tierney activities of living model; the Orem self-care model; and King's theory of goal attainment.
3. Define a therapeutic relationship and describe its benefits to patients.
4. Discuss patient-centred care in the context of medical and veterinary healthcare.
5. Recognise the principles of multidisciplinary teamworking within the veterinary profession.

The nursing profession is diverse and, considering both veterinary and human centred nursing as a whole, the scope of practice is huge. From endoscopy to oncology, anaesthesia support to wound care, the skill set varies immensely. In veterinary nursing, this is emphasised by the need to nurse different species, which demands further specific skills and knowledge.

Despite considerable differences in roles and responsibilities, nurses share a focus and approach. It might be assumed that regardless of what department in the hospital a nurse works, or which species of animal they are treating, a nurse will have the needs of their patient at the front of their mind. Every nurse can rely on the nursing process or veterinary nursing process to guide their thought and help them plan appropriate care.

The nursing process provides a problem-solving method to apply to a situation. It is a tool that can be used by nurses to structure their approach to patient care. It doesn't actually provide any detail for what needs to be done. It explains that an assessment of a patient must be performed, but gives no detail as to what questions should be asked or where the emphasis should be placed. It instructs care planning, but gives no detail as to how to carry it out.

Models of nursing fill those gaps in the nursing process. Walsh [1] describes this succinctly with the nursing process as a tool to provide structure to care delivery and models of nursing care as tools to instruct on how care should be given.

Models of nursing have two main functions for nurses in practice. First, they can offer a range of beliefs and values to guide nurses through the stages of the nursing process and provide direction on what is important and relevant. Models offer a philosophy of nursing.

Second, nursing models may include very specific directions on what assessments should be carried out and how. They include specific lists of body systems or patient needs that should be considered during the care process, aiming to promote a holistic approach to care. Looking back to the origins of nursing, Florence Nightingale's model of care was very much about controlling the environment of the patient to allow nature to cure the patient. Today, the priorities of care are different and the models used represent these changes. There are a range of different beliefs, values, and priorities that might be encountered on a daily basis in practice.

To illustrate the use of nursing models, they may be applied to an everyday activity, like buying a new house. It is easy to link the nursing process into the process of buying a house. A family plans to move, so they assess where to live and what sort of facilities they would like. The process is planned, the family visits estate agents or looks online. The intervention happens when the family moves in and then evaluation is continuous as the family lives in the house, decorates it, assesses it, and possibly moves out as their circumstances or needs change.

This is a fairly standard process. However, estate agents will all understand that different groups of people are likely to place their emphasis on different priorities. So, a young family with children will need to prioritise access to schools. An older couple looking to downsize from the family home will often look for amenities close by. A young professional couple with no children might put services such as restaurants, shops and entertainment venues high on their list.

So, each estate agent cannot treat each family the same, despite the fact that they all need to buy a new house.

It is the same with nursing. Most patients need care to make them feel better as a primitive and basic requirement. However, the priorities that the patient have vary considerably. The type of care they need varies and models of care provide guidance to ensure patient needs are met and the correct care is planned and implemented.

Nursing models in practice

Consider Jim, a seven-year-old Doberman admitted after being hit by a car, with a fractured femur and a ruptured diaphragm. This patient needs help and support in most of his care needs. The model of nursing requires the nurse to assist with and potentially take over some of his physiological systems with respiratory support, administration of drugs, comprehensive analgesia and wound care.

In contrast, Simon is a newly diagnosed diabetic cat who requires a different type of nursing. Once stabilised Simon requires ongoing support and medication from his owner. Owner education is the priority and the model of care needs to emphasise the use of effective communication skills to develop a relationship with Simon's owner.

Mona is a young female cat coming into the practice for neutering and needs a different model of care again. She is not unwell and so her self-care, eating, grooming and exercising should be supported before and after the routine procedure. This model of care involves an intervention and a swift return to health so that Mona can return to her home environment as soon as possible.

The cases above demonstrate nursing care, with different priorities, values and ideas behind the actions. They demonstrate an acute care model, a care partnership model, and health promotion model.

Roper, Logan and Tierney activities of living model

There are established nursing models that can be examined and potentially borrowed from human-centred nursing and adapted to use in veterinary nursing. Probably one of the most well-known is the Roper, Logan and Tierney (RLT) Activities of Living Model [2]. The original foundations of this model were published in the 1983 book written by Nancy Roper. This model is used frequently throughout the NHS and its associated 12 activities of living (ALs) are often used as a format or template for patient admission documents.

The emphasis of the RLT Activities of Living Model was to move away from medical, disease-based nursing work and encourage consideration of the person as a whole. The RLT model uses five key themes to model nursing care, the 12 ALs, a group of five factors identified as having an influence on the ALs factors, the lifespan of the patient, a dependence-independence continuum and patient individuality (Figure 3.1).

Activities of living

The first theme for this model is helping people to prevent, alleviate, solve or cope with actual problems and potential problems associated with the activities of living. The plan of nursing care is then linked through to goals of care produced from assessing the patient's ability to carry out the 12 ALs. RLT were clear in their emphasis on assessing rather than assessment, demonstrating the need for continuous evaluation of care.

So, in a two-part process, a full patient assessment is made where the baseline ability to carry out ALs can be assessed. Then, a further assessment of any altered ALs that mean the patient will require assistance are identified, including the acknowledgment of potential problems as well as actual ones.

Roper, Logan and Tierney cite a series of factors that may affect a person's ALs which emphasise and account for the individuality of a patient's needs. Alongside the biological factors

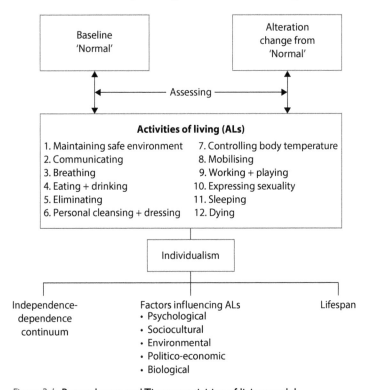

Figure 3.1 **Roper, Logan and Tierney activities of living model.**

usually accounted for in the patient's health status, they highlight that psychological, sociocultural, environmental and politico-economic factors will all influence the patient and the care they need. The term sociocultural is a combination of consideration of social and cultural factors. This incorporates the lifestyle and values of people, their religion, attitudes, experiences and economic status. Psychological factors take into account the mind of the patient. The way they think, the way they subsequently behave, their character, disposition, demeanour and temperament. Politico-economic factors encourage nurses to think widely about their patient, the attitudes and beliefs they may hold and how that may apply to their health status. Economic factors are also relevant to nursing care, ranging from the costs associated with being ill, managing a restricted income through being off work to attend appointments, to patients accessing private healthcare and dealing with associated costs.

The model uses an independence continuum. It encourages nurses to take into account the assistance that may be needed for a patient to achieve their ALs. This links directly with the evaluation of a patient's care. Goals can be set to achieve a reduction in the level of assistance. This factor also demonstrates the importance of establishing a patient's 'normal' during an assessment so that nurses understand the level of independence a person had at home before they were unwell and goals may be set accordingly.

The fourth theme in this model acknowledges the life stage of the patient, highlighting eight key developmental stages all influencing what patients can and can't do. They are all linked through to each AL and how the patient can be helped to carry it out. So, in veterinary nursing, consideration of the age of the patient may lead to an adjustment in facilities to support elimination, for example, a lower sided tray for an elderly arthritic cat or assisted elimination for neonates. The combination of consideration of patient's age or their relative dependence on another to fulfil their ALs also contributes to an individualised patient assessment.

Applying Roper, Logan and Tierney's activities of living model to veterinary nursing

This model is readily adapted to animals. Its clear structure facilitates an easy-to-follow assessment protocol, stimulating consideration of the individual needs of patients to ensure they are able to carry out their activities of living.

Breathing, eliminating and maintaining body temperature

Physiologically, there are three activities of living that apply directly to animals: breathing, eliminating and maintaining body temperature. Here the key point is that even though all animals will share these needs, highlighting them as part of an assessment process raises the awareness of the individuality of these shared needs. Therefore, all cats must urinate, however, individual habits mean that different facilities must be provided to support that. Potentially different litter tray substrates, for example, the use of earth from the garden to replicate outside urination, could help encourage cats to use a litter tray.

Sleeping

This activity of living is an example of extrapolating evidence from human-centred nursing, which places an emphasis on sleep and its restorative properties. It is easy to extrapolate this to animals and set routines within the hospital environment to support sleep. Individualistic factors also apply; an anxious dog might sleep better in an enclosed bed. Lights can be turned off to replicate the normal routine to encourage rest and recuperation.

Mobilising

Consideration of mobilisation for animals is important. Pressure area care within human health is an area of intense focus and funding. Improved training staff and the increased use of assessment tools has raised awareness and highlighted the need for proactive work to prevent pressure damage in less mobile patients.

Supported mobilisation may improve recovery and recuperation of orthopaedic injuries or facilitate clear breathing as an animal is propped up in an upright sternal position as opposed to lying laterally. Consideration of the influencing factors advocated by Roper, Logan and Tierney may facilitate a greater depth of assessment; providing a suitable environment with supportive equipment may facilitate rehabilitation through assisted movement to increase strength. However, if this environment cannot be replicated at home because the owner doesn't have the strength or facilities, further hospitalisation may be indicated.

Cleaning and dressing

Clearly dressing is not necessarily relevant to animals but, in a direct extrapolation, rugs for horses may be part of routine nursing care. Dressings and bandages protecting surgical sites need to be comfortable to prevent animals removing them. Cleaning and personal hygiene is part of making a patient comfortable as well as preventing problems such as urine scalding or other skin irritation. Cleaning the faces of kittens with cat flu may facilitate vision and a clear nasal passageway so that they are more likely to eat as they can smell the food available to them.

Communication

In this case, this AL may be applied to the direct communication animals have with their carers through subtle behavioural hints and clues that can be interpreted to judge how to approach them and how to minimise stress and anxiety.

Alternatively, this AL may be adapted to consider the communication between the patient's carer and the veterinary healthcare professional. Without the knowledge, understanding and support of a patient's carer, it is unlikely that any medical treatment will produce positive results. It links directly to the sociocultural factors mentioned by RLT as communicating with owners can be complex. Some owners will have preconceived ideas on how the patient may be treated which might be challenging to overcome.

Sexuality

With animals, this can be directly linked to the relevant life stage. At a lower life stage, neutering might be indicated for pets. This is for health promotion and also for development of the animal–human relationship, which might be facilitated through neutering, as unpleasant marking should stop and the need to seek a mate dissipates, reducing the likelihood of running away.

Consideration of the neutering state of an animal might also link to the prevention of specific health problems, such as testicular tumours or pyometra.

Working and playing

This is relevant for animals that seek the company of humans; pets will often enjoy human company, even when unwell. Furthermore, any positive attention that a member of the veterinary healthcare team can provide may offset the unpleasant procedure that has just occurred and facilitate further treatment. Marking a care plan when an animal last received friendly attention, kindness, or play (often referred to as TLC – tender loving care) can potentially help plan future interventions and help decide when they should be carried out.

In addition, vet nurses shouldn't be too quick to dismiss the 'working' aspect of this activity of living. Working animals are part of our lives and returning an animal back to health may be a key goal of treatment. Potentially, the likelihood of it being able to return to work may even influence whether treatment is supported or not.

Eating and drinking, maintaining a safe environment and dying

Considered together, these activities of daily living for animals are linked; they are all controlled almost entirely by human contact. These are factors linked through to the independence continuum emphasised by RLT. While farm animals may seek feed across the countryside, during cold winters they rely on supplemental feeding and care from professionals. Pets are almost entirely dependent on carers for feeding, particularly if kept indoors. It is these ALs that highlight the need for carer/owner communication and education from nurses to facilitate the best care for the animal. For without owner education and communication, dependant animals will not receive the care they need.

It is clear that the RLT model may be usefully applied to veterinary nursing, and may provide a clear and detailed structure to assess a patient. Nancy Roper was clear in her assertions that the model must not become a simplistic checklist. In veterinary nursing, it is necessary that each AL is considered within the context of that animal and their actual or potential problem. If the activity of daily living is simply checked off as something that the patient can or can't do, a tick box exercise, key aspects of care might be missed. Where would pain or anxiety be addressed? There is a need to ensure nurses look deeper and use the factors described by RLT; the sociocultural, politico-economic, psychological, biological and environmental factors. In doing so, nurses will be able to start to understand why an animal is unable to carry out a particular AL. They can then ask, is it pain that is stopping the animal? Trauma? Behaviour problems? Limited resources?

Sociocultural

Sociocultural factors will influence the patient, most commonly via the attitudes and understanding of their owner. An owner's beliefs and culture may facilitate a particular treatment option, some cultures have limited empathy for pet-keeping, so advanced veterinary treatments may not be considered.

Politico-economic

The most obvious influencing factor acting on veterinary health care is that of finances. Challenges may occur between what the owner can afford and what the veterinary nurse or vet sees as the best treatment plan. While the animal's health and welfare must always be the primary consideration, reassessment and compromise is required to optimise patient care within the confines of the budget available.

Environmental

The influence of the owner is highlighted further when considering environmental factors that might affect the animal. This ranges from the physical location of where the animal lives, whether it is clean and safe, to the environmental influences that may affect the animal, such as passive smoking, the opportunity to rifle through dustbins and eat inappropriate food, or living with fear from an aggressive owner.

Psychology

Psychological care is just as important with animals, many owners seek advice for their animal's behavioural problems and some behavioural problems might be solved through addressing physical problems. It is another relevant factor to consider, as it may affect the healthcare of an animal.

Knowledge of each of these influencing factors is useful. They should exist as a line of thought alongside the activities of daily living, encouraging nurses to liaise with the patient owners, talk concepts through and ensure that mutual goals are set within the boundaries produced by consideration of these factors.

When it comes to veterinary nursing, however, a disadvantage with RLT is the emphasis it puts on the patient. While this is advantageous when dealing with human patients, it ignores the key element of working with animals, the need to work with their owners. Reflecting on the definitions of nursing discussed in chapter one, the paediatric definition of nursing illustrates that care must be family-centred, not just patient-centred, due to the age of the patient. Veterinary nursing is the same, not due to the age of the patient, but simply due to the species difference. Any nursing model must incorporate consideration of the owner of the animal.

King's theory of goal attainment

King's model of nursing [3], her theory of goal attainment, incorporates consideration of the support network for a patient. Developed in 1971 by Imogen King, it is a more conceptual model when compared to the descriptive and instructional RLT model, which provides a practical approach to care delivery. The aim of King's model is to create purposeful interactions to set mutual goals and agree on the means to achieve the goals. In human-centred nursing, the emphasis is clearly on the relationship between the nurse and the patient. However, in veterinary nursing, this may be adapted to emphasise the development of a therapeutic relationship between the nurse and the patient's owner.

Put simply, **a therapeutic relationship** within veterinary nursing is one that is an interaction, between nurse and the owner of the patient, that is beneficial to the health of the patient. In human-centred nursing, it will involve clear lines of communication. The nurse needs to try and demonstrate care and empathy for the patient and an interest in them as an individual to facilitate a two-way process of mutual respect so that care plans may be developed and implemented collaboratively.

This model, which emphasises the therapeutic relationship, is possibly more relevant to human and veterinary healthcare in 2017 than it was when it was initially discussed in the 1970s.

There are three main reasons why King's model should be considered a relevant model of nursing in today's healthcare system.

1. Increased co-morbidities/increased longevity of life
2. Shift in culture of healthcare from the paternalistic, medical model to a holistic, patient-centred care model
3. Multidisciplinary teamworking

Co-morbidities

It is well-documented that patients are now living longer, often with multiple chronic healthcare problems. This results in longer term care needs and repeated interactions with healthcare professionals. Effective communication is the cornerstone to developing a therapeutic relationship and this model emphasises the need for clear and coherent communication skills.

This model of care can be replicated in animals. Clinically, the patient demographics for animals echo those of the human-centred world. Animals are living longer and nurses are routinely supporting owners to care for patients at home with long-term health problems such as renal failure, diabetes or cancers. There are more options for the care of these chronically ill patients and with that comes the need for longer term support from the veterinary team. To care for these animals and ensure their needs are met, the emphasis must be on the relationship with the owner of the animal as they will be the people providing direct care through medication, diet and monitoring. King emphasises the need for mutual goal setting, so both parties are aware of the aims and potential outcomes of treatment which should improve the likelihood of achieving positive outcomes.

Patient-centred care

Historically, human-centred healthcare has adopted a paternalistic model of care. Paternalistic healthcare is when healthcare professionals exert full authority over their patients. Medical decisions will be made exclusively by the professional team. Healthcare becomes something that is done to the patient, rather than with the patient.

Recently this model has been challenged and there is a cultural shift towards a patient-centred approach to healthcare. **Patient-centred care** moves care decision-making to the patient with the involvement of their families and their carers. It alters the role of the healthcare professional, for instead of making decisions on behalf of the patient, they must take steps to support the patient's decision-making process, perhaps through teaching or counselling. Patient-centred care and holistic care are terms that are often used interchangeably, however they are quite separate. Holistic care is care that aims to incorporate all patient needs, rather than focusing on their problem area. It reminds nursing staff that aspects of a patient's mental health or social situation may have an impact on their health and so may become part of their care needs. Patient-centred care is an emphasis on ensuring the patient's choices and opinions are always taken into account throughout their care journey.

The principles of patient-centred care coincide with working with a general public who are increasingly more knowledgeable about healthcare. **Health literacy,** which may be defined as the cognitive and social resources needed for individuals and communities to access, understand and use information and services to make decisions about healthcare is increasing. The use of the Internet and social media, television and radio make for a population who have higher levels of health literacy and therefore are more likely to be able to engage in decision making.

In the UK, this shift in culture is supported through the NHS constitution [4], which states, 'The patient will be at the heart of everything the NHS does. It should support individuals to promote and manage their own health. Patients, with their families and carers, where appropriate, will be involved in and consulted on all decisions about their care and treatment'.

The emphasis that King's model of care puts on planning and goal setting supports this patient-centred model of care. It puts collaborative working between the professional and the patient at the heart of planning care. The care plan almost becomes a contract, an agreed plan of action with interventions to be performed by both patient and professional.

This shift in human-centred healthcare may also be extrapolated to veterinary healthcare. Patient-centred care in veterinary nursing may be interpreted as making a direct connection with the owners of the animal. Instead of simply telling them what to do with their animal, opportunities should be taken to create a dialogue, a relationship, one that facilitates their understanding and produces goals for the care of the animal.

Multidisciplinary teamworking

King's model of care promotes inter-professional communication. It encourages collaboration, supporting the creation of joint care goals with agreed methods of achieving those goals. This supports the professional obligation that both human and animal centred healthcare team members have to develop clear lines of communication with colleagues to support continuity of care and patient safety.

Patient care in the veterinary profession may often be spread out between practices, particularly in an emergency. Care outside of office hours may be given at a different clinic to routine healthcare. The teams will all have the same goals, to achieve optimum health for the patient. However, they may have different means to achieve it, which could potentially lead to conflict and poor patient care.

Consider a patient admitted to an emergency clinic after a traffic accident. The emergency vet places a central venous catheter and administers a constant rate infusion of analgesia. While this

In practice – Multidisciplinary team working

Bart is a seven-year-old terrier who has just undergone a cruciate repair. Initially his post-operative care is provided by the veterinary surgeon and the veterinary nurse. A weight management programme through appropriate diet selection combined with anti-inflammatory and analgesic medication is instigated. Several weeks after his procedure, Bart's post-operative recovery is complicated by the fact that Bart refuses to use the affected leg and runs happily along on three legs. The operation was a success and x-rays are normal. However, Bart continues to run on three legs. Bart is referred for hydrotherapy to encourage him to use his hind leg. Direct contact between the veterinary surgeon, nurse, and physiotherapist is essential to facilitate a comprehensive, multidisciplinary plan of care to achieve shared goals. The most common way of receiving information about patients being seen by other members of the MDT (multidisciplinary team) is through letter, however more often email may facilitate swift and efficient referrals. The inclusion of the goals of care in the documentation enables all team members to plan their therapy accordingly.

benefits the patient in that moment, when it comes to 8 am and the care is to be handed over to the daytime practice where staff are not trained in managing central venous catheters, suddenly the patient is more vulnerable. Even though the goals are the same, it cannot be assumed that the methods of achieving those goals will be the same, and clear and open communication is needed to ensure mutually agreeable methods are being used.

Interestingly, one of the key criticisms of King's model in human-centred nursing is the impracticality of its use for patients that have limited ability to communicate with their nurse. Its emphasis on setting goals with the patient is considered an obstruction to its use with certain patient groups. Paradoxically, it is this emphasis which suits veterinary nursing. Obviously setting goals with animal patients is not practical, however, if the emphasis is switched wholly to setting goals with the patient's owner, the model applies well. So, while King's model doesn't describe how to assess a patient, or what details to think about, it provides a clear emphasis on communication that will facilitate effective patient care.

Orem's model of self-care

In human-centred nursing, Orem's model of care [5] is based on the assumption that people are able to look after themselves. However, to do so, they require resources, information, skills and motivation. If a patient becomes unwell, it may be assumed that they lack the ability to self-care, as they have lost the resources, information, skills or motivation. Orem describes this as a self-care deficit. The self-care deficit is an equivalent to the actual or potential problems as identified by the RLT model. When this self-deficit becomes bigger than the ability to self-care, nursing is required. Orem believed that in order to stay healthy there are eight basic needs that have to be met, called universal self-care requisites (USCR's).

Orem's universal self care needs

1. Sufficient intake of air
2. Sufficient intake of water
3. Sufficient intake of food
4. Satisfactory eliminative functions
5. Activity balanced with rest
6. Balance between solitude and social interaction
7. Prevention of hazards to life, human functions and human well being
8. Promotion of human functioning and development within social groups in accordance with human potential, the desire for normalcy

These are more generalised than the RLT activities of daily living, but use the same principle of providing detail to the assessment stage of the nursing process. The most relevant emphasis of the Orem model for veterinary nursing is the need to understand how the patient usually cares for themselves, so the concept of normalcy for that patient. It describes the nurse as taking on one of six roles to support that recovery of the patient to enable them to self-care. In veterinary nursing, the initial goal may well be to facilitate the transition of care from the veterinary team to the owner, and then eventually to the patient when they become independent.

Six roles of nursing or helping a patient

1. Doing for or acting for another
2. Guiding or directing another
3. Providing physical support
4. Providing psychological support
5. Providing an environment supportive of development
6. Teaching another

In practice – Orem's self-care model

Hermann is a 10-year-old Dutch warmblood horse and presented with a de-gloving injury on his foreleg. Initially the veterinary team must take on the role of **acting for** the patient and providing physical support for the wound through cleaning and surgery. The next step in the process, once the wound has been attended to under general anaesthetic and appropriate medication administered, is for the team to act as a **guide for the owner** so they can take their horse home and continue to administer the medication they require to **support** the healing of the wound. Once the medication is finished, the only remaining stage is a truly self-caring stage, where the animal's own physiology takes over and heals the wound entirely.

Any model that is used in healthcare, be it medical or veterinary, must be relevant and useful to that specific field. King's, Orem's and the RLT models may be adapted to veterinary nursing. In discussing these models, this chapter on touches on their main themes and key emphasis. The original texts are still available and reading them will provide a more in depth understanding of the principles the authors wanted to apply.

Adaptation of the language of a model might well be indicated when transferring a model of care from human beings to animals. Once in place, the model should be practiced and used with the relevant patients. It may be tempting to adapt the model further and leave out parts of the model or assessment process that seem irrelevant to the patient's presenting situation. However, that would result in a return to the medical model as care would be concentrated purely on the contemporary symptoms and not the whole patient. Using a model should ensure that all patient needs are met, so once selected it should be used in its entirety.

Review

- Nursing models represent the way care should be carried out, the model of care that is used may be determined by the context of the care, emergency versus chronic illness versus health promotion.
- Models of care can provide detail to the nursing process by providing an explicit framework on which to structure an assessment, a plan of care and an evaluation.
- Patient-centred care requires nursing staff to support patients to make decisions about their healthcare. This is a model of care that is likely to extend into veterinary nursing with an emphasis on the development of a therapeutic relationship between owner and nurse.
- Effective communication between members of the multidisciplinary team and patient owners may be supported by the use of nursing models within the nursing process.

Further reflections

Many human-centred nursing models promote an emphasis on self-care. Given that animals rely on humans to fulfil many of their basic care needs, are such models really useful tools to provide a foundation of veterinary nursing theory? Additionally, several models emphasise the need for a therapeutic relationship, and when this is applied to veterinary nursing, this emphasis may be extrapolated to the relationship between the veterinary nursing and the patient's owner. However, is it possible to develop a therapeutic relationship directly between an animal and their nurse? What sort of characteristics would that relationship have? What lines of communication might be used? If it were possible, how would facilitation of such a relationship benefit the patient? Could any benefits be measured objectively?

References

1. Walsh M (2002). *Models and Critical Pathways in Clinical Nursing.* 2nd ed. Edinburgh: Bailliere Tindall.
2. Roper N, Logan WW, and Tierney AJ (1996). *The Elements of Nursing.* 4th ed. Edinburgh: Churchill Livingstone.
3. King IM (1981). *A Theory for Nursing: Systems, Concepts, Process.* New York, NY: John Wiley & Sons.
4. The NHS Constition [online]. Last accessed 27th March 2017. https://www.gov.uk/government/uploads/system/uploads/attachment_data/file/480482/NHS_Constitution_WEB.pdf.
5. Orem DE (2001). *Nursing: Concepts of Practice.* 5th ed. St Louis, MO: CV Mosby.

Further reading

This book offers a greater insight into the work of nursing theorists.

1. *Nursing Theorists and Their Work*, 8th edition. Martha Raile Aligood (Mosby, 2013).

Chapter 4

Holistic care in veterinary nursing

By the end of this chapter you will be able to

1. Identify the principles of the Orpet and Jeffery Ability Model of care.
2. List the 10 abilities as established in the Ability Model of care.
3. Define culture in relation to how an owner may influence a patient's care plan.
4. Discuss the principles of owner compliance and its impact on patient care and care planning.
5. Describe how models of care, combined with the veterinary nursing process, facilitate nursing care plans.

Promoting holistic care

In 2006, there was a change in the way that veterinary nursing was taught in the United Kingdom. Nursing models and care plans were introduced to the syllabus and there was a move away from traditional teaching, which involved addressing an illness or condition individually, listing pathogenesis, clinical sign, diagnostic tool, and treatment option. Instead, students were taught how to correctly identify clinical signs and symptoms, prioritise the care required, understand pathophysiology, and implement the appropriate nursing intervention. Student veterinary nurses were being encouraged to think laterally, to approach a patient as a whole, and use the nursing process.

These ideas were promoted through the much-cited articles from Hilary Orpet and Andrea Jeffery, published in the *Veterinary Nursing Journal* in 2006. They outlined the movement away from the medical model of care towards holistic assessment and use of the problem-solving approach to nursing through use of assessment, planning, implementation and evaluation.

In Practice – Medical vs holistic approach to care of feline diabetic patient

Medical model

Pathogenesis

A complex disorder of carbohydrate, fat and protein metabolism that is primarily a result of a deficiency or complete lack of insulin secretion by the beta cells of the pancreas or resistance to insulin.

Clinical signs

Polyuria
Polydipsia
Weight loss

Diagnosis

Blood tests
Urinalysis

Treatment options

Injection of insulin twice daily
Modification of diet

Plan

Owner to inject insulin twice daily
Feed specific diabetic cat food

Holistic nursing care model

History

Six-year-old domestic short hair cat called Butch presents to veterinary practice with inappropriate urination on furniture and bedding. On examination, weight loss is noted since the last visit to the veterinary practice. No other abnormalities are detected.
Urinalysis demonstrates glucosuria.
Blood tests demonstrate hyperglycaemia, dehydration, and mild electrolyte imbalance.
Owner works full time and cares for elderly parents – Butch is fully insured.
Owner happy to use twice daily insulin to manage symptoms, but nervous of the amount of appointments the cat will need in the future, as they may struggle with making time to bring the cat to the vet.

Plan

Admit for stabilisation and intravenous fluid therapy to address dehydration and electrolyte imbalance.
Nursing care plan designed to support owner education on injection technique.
Step by step instructions written for owner to gradually transfer Butch onto diabetic diet from his regular food.
Follow up phone call appointments are made over the next three days with a face to face appointment in five days' time.

Reflection and learning

Butch has polyuria and polydipsia caused by glucosuria which upsets electrolyte balance causing diuresis, hence inappropriate urination when Butch did not have access to outside.
Diabetes is caused by a resistance to or lack of insulin from the beta cells of the pancreas, hence the need for supplementation through injections.

The Orpet and Jeffery Ability Model 2007

In 2007, at the annual British Small Animal Veterinary Association congress, Orpet and Jeffery introduced their novel Ability Model of nursing [1], specifically designed for veterinary nursing (Figure 4.1). Just like the human-centred nursing theorists from the 1960s and 1970s, their aim was to design a model of care that encouraged veterinary nurses to move away from a medical model and embrace the holistic approach. They wanted to encourage the very best care for animals in veterinary practices. Their work coincided with changes to national animal welfare legislation with the introduction of the Animal Welfare Act 2006 [2] which made owners and those temporarily responsible for an animal legally responsible to ensure that five needs of welfare for animals under their care were met.

Animal Welfare Act 2006 – Five needs of welfare

- Need for a suitable environment
- Need for a suitable diet
- Need to be able to exhibit normal behaviour patterns
- Need to be housed with, or apart, from other animals
- Need to be protected from pain, suffering, injury and disease

Orpet and Jeffery were influenced by Orem and Roper, Logan and Tierney's (RLT) models of care in their design of the Ability Model. Nursing models can provide a set of values to guide nurses through the problem solving process and provide direction on what is important. Additionally, they can also explicitly describe what assessments should be taken and when. The Ability Model fulfils both those functions. It provides explicit detail for veterinary nurses assessing patients and provides a set of values and beliefs. It moves the veterinary nurse away from

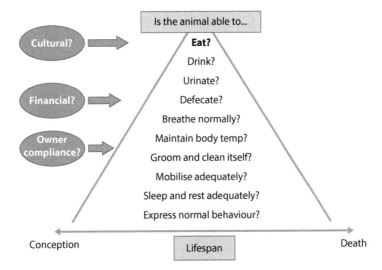

Figure 4.1 Ability Model. (From Orpet H and Welsh P: *Handbook of Veterinary Nursing.* 2011. Copyright Wiley-VCH Verlag GmbH & Co. KGaA. Reproduced with permission.)

simply providing medical treatments at the direction of the veterinary surgeon, to a process of developing their own assessment and gathering nursing-specific information from both the animal and their owner.

The Ability Model begins with an assessment stage where both subjective and objective information is collected. The assessment is centred on 10 abilities and the priority is to establish what is normal for the individual patient. The 10 abilities were identified as the fundamental elements an animal requires to function and demonstrate normal behaviour.

The Ability Model advocates the use of a questionnaire with the owners of animals, based on the 10 abilities. The model encourages VNs to understand the normal care and routine of a patient, so that an environment might be created for the animal that minimises stress through integration of as many of their normal husbandry practices as possible.

While interviewing and speaking to the owner's communication style is important, and to gather the appropriate level of detailed information, open-ended questions are suggested. These are questions that require a descriptive answer from the owner, based on their knowledge and emotions. This is in contrast to closed questions, which require a simple yes or no answer.

Consider if an owner is asked whether their cat eats twice a day; a simple answer of yes provides reassurance that the cat is eating but provides absolutely no detail. Asking for more detail helps the nursing team provide a more suitable environment for the animal. Nurses must not make assumptions; an animal may well be eating, but potentially not eating the correct food, or not eating enough. Asking what the cat's eating habits are is more open ended and invites more detail. Owners in need of encouragement may be prompted further with direct, factual questions. The nurse may ask what time the animal eats, what they eat, or what bowls they use and what their favourite foods are. Instigating such a conversation with an owner may well stimulate them to offer additional information that they might not have considered important before. The aim is to establish any inabilities the animal has, or has the potential to have, so that care interventions may be put into place to prevent them or solve them (Figure 4.2).

The Ability Model should be considered in conjunction with the veterinary nursing process, with prioritisation running through it. VNs should take time to consider the abilities listed in the Ability Model and think through which are the most important to address first. The model suggests that VNs ask, is the animal able to....? While all abilities should be assessed, some will need more urgent attention than others. Methodical assessment is advocated. It is clear that some animals are not going to tolerate a full examination until they have received analgesia and started to recover from the initial physical and psychological shock of being involved in whatever problem has befallen them (Figure 4.3).

The process of writing down each intervention required to address any problems with an ability is what makes up a care plan. In addition, the goal of the intervention may also be recorded on the care plan to assist evaluation and monitoring of progress. Once each intervention is carried out, it can be marked off on the care plan, providing a record of the care given which may then have extended uses throughout the practice and indeed the veterinary nursing profession.

The evaluation stage of the process is guided, once again, by the 10 abilities. Each ability is reassessed to understand whether the animal has changed in the level of care it requires. It is clear to see how the Ability Model provides the detail for the stages of the nursing process as RLT did for human nursing. The abilities are a clear checklist of elements to address in the animal to ensure its comfort and functionality. As with human-centred nursing, the use of a model of care within the nursing process allows for an individualised plan of care to be put together. While conditions of health may be similar, there are external factors that can individualise how an animal may be treated by the veterinary team.

Help us get to know your pet better so we can make
their stay with us as comfortable as possible.

Name of pet *Ruby*   Your surname *Simpson*

What does your pet normally eat? *Dry dog biscuits.*

Does he/she have a favourite food? *She will eat anything!*

Dose he/she have any particular eating habits? *Stealing from my
young son – She loves human food.*

How does your pet usually drink water? *From a bowl in the house.*

What are your pets usual toilet habits? *Uses garden (grass) or on walk.*

Does your pet have any breathing problems? *No.*
If yes, what makes them worse?
If yes, what makes them better?

Can your pet groom themselves independently? *Yes.*

Where does your pet sleep usually? *On my bed.*

Is there anything your pet particularly likes or dislikes?
*Loves walks and sleeping on sofa, and enjoys company of people.
Doesn't like loud noises.*

Does your pet take medication easily? *Yes – with cheese.*
If not, how do you normally administer medication?

Please note any further information you think might be helpful below.
Ruby often barks when strangers come to the house or pass me on a walk.

Figure 4.2 **In practice – The use of an owner questionnaire to
establish normal health status and routine husbandry
of a patient.**

Individualised care needs

In human-centred nursing, Roper, Logan and Tierney listed these factors as biological, psycho-logical, environmental, sociocultural and politico-economic. Orpet and Jeffery follow a similar pattern, listing culture, finance and owner compliance as the three key factors that will affect the care given to an animal.

The consideration of these of factors is particularly important in the care of veterinary patients, as it might be argued that not many animals coming into the veterinary hospital are self-caring. So, while an assessment may concentrate on what is perceived they are able to do independently, they rely on the veterinary team and their owners for the care. While they may be able to eat independently, they can only do so if food is provided for them. It is this aspect that reinforces the need for an effective relationship between nurse and owner to ensure that care can be given. Clear education and advice is required, and links back into the consideration of family-centred care that paediatric nurses advocate where the child and its family are at the centre of the care. This empha-sis demonstrates the importance of a therapeutic relationship with the owner. It has potential

Example of completed assessment after discussing with owner

NAME	Dolly	
BREED	JRT	
AGE	8 years	
HX	Mitral valve disease-medical management	
CURRENT DIAGNOSIS	Congestive HF Pulmonary oedema	

ASSESSMENT Is the animal able to	HOME/NORMAL	CURRENT
1. Eat?	Yes – eats dry food only	Limited due to dyspnoea
2. Drink?	Yes	Limited due to dyspnoea
3. Urinate?	Yes – on grass	Yes – diuretics likely to urinate more
4. Defecate?	Yes – on grass (not usually in garden)	No concerns
5. Breathe normally	Yes – but exercise tolerance has ↓	Not currently on O_2 therapy
6. Maintain body temp?	Yes	Requires monitoring when possible as in O_2 cape
7. Groom + clean itself?	Yes – does not like being brushed at all	Limited due to dyspnoea
8. Mobilise adequately?	Yes – loves walks, does agility classes	Poor due to dyspnoea, propped up in sternal to expand chest breathing
9. Sleep + rest adequately?	Yes – has a bed in kitchen	Yes
10. Express normal behaviours	Yes	Limited due to dyspnoea

NOTES FROM OWNER – not good at taking tablets – spits them out, won't eat them in food/guards left hindlimb sometimes (arthritis) and may snap

Figure 4.3 In practice – The use of the Ability Model to assess a dog admitted with congestive heart failure.

implications for the development of the role of veterinary nursing as more and more VNs take on health promotion and chronic care roles alongside delivering acute care. Like Roper, Logan and Tierney, Orpet and Jeffery highlight the lifespan of the patient as part of their model, as a timeline, from conception to death. This is a crucial reminder of a characteristic of the patient that will contribute to the need for individual care. The age of the patient should be taken into account. While an older cat might be relied upon to ignore an intravenous catheter in its foreleg, a four-month-old kitten, with his naturally inquisitive nature, cannot be relied upon in the same way.

Nursing care may then be adapted accordingly; the elderly cat may appreciate time out of its kennel curled up on the nurse's lap. However, the eight-month-old kitten is unlikely to settle in such a way and is more likely to want attention and stimulus through playing with toys.

Culture, finance and compliance

Culture, finance and owner compliance are all deeply relevant to veterinary nursing and how any veterinary nurse may plan the care of an animal. Culturally, there are many different attitudes to animals. The culture of an owner will depend on their experiences, their lifestyle, customs and education. While the human-animal bond may be extremely strong in some people, others rely on their animals for working and may be entirely pragmatic about their animal's health and wellbeing. So, a sheep dog with a questionable working future due to ill health may be provided with rudimentary care to facilitate functionality or euthanised if there is no prospect of it returning to work. In comparison, a family pet suffering a similar injury might well be referred for expert veterinary attention, the primary goal of care being to return the healthy pet to its family.

Financially, the differences are obvious. Veterinary healthcare receives no government funding and not all owners of animals have the ability to pay for the treatment required. Care plans may need to be modified to reduce costs or again, euthanasia might be an option should owners be unable to finance any care at all.

Owner compliance is a key part of any planned care. Patients are often cared for at home through the use of medication and/or specific diets. Options are often available should owners be unable to facilitate care. Animals may have extended stays in veterinary hospitals, care plans might be modified so that medication administration is minimised, or owners might be trained by veterinary nurses to administer medication and care safely and accurately.

Each of these factors must be considered when care is being planned. There is no point in developing a potentially long and complex wound care plan that involves multiple visits to the veterinary hospital when an owner can afford neither the costs nor the time involved to care for the animal. So, while veterinary nurses can be trained to develop care plans of a high quality with individual care for each animal, such care plans are of little consequence if not considered in conjunction with the financial, cultural and compliance factors.

The Ability Model is a clear and easy to use model of care for veterinary nursing. It promotes a structured way of thinking through the use of the nursing process. It helps VNs to ensure they are providing holistic care and therefore, do not leave out elements of care that are just as essential but easily missed in the face of more pressing demands during periods of ill health.

Furthermore, an additional, significant advantage of using such a model of care is the increased interaction that is stimulated through the owner questionnaire. If the questionnaire is carried out in a face to face interview, the owner and the nurse get a chance to begin to build up a relationship which ultimately should benefit the care of the patient in question.

Review

- The Ability Model advocates consideration of a list of 10 activities; life span of the animal; and the culture, compliance and financial situation of the patient's owner.
- Using a questionnaire with the owner of an animal being admitted to veterinary care can provide useful information to support the care of the patient in practice, as well as providing a useful baseline for comparison and goal setting.
- The communication style used by the veterinary nurse has a large influence on the quantity and quality of information that may be provided by an owner.
- Holistic care involves taking into account all the patient's needs, not just those which are altered through ill health.

Further reflections

A nursing colleague comes to you to ask about Orpet and Jeffery's Ability Model of care. They have applied it to a patient who has recently been admitted following a trauma. They are confused as to where certain aspects of the patient's assessment fits within the Ability Model. Specifically, they ask you where pain relief, cardiovascular measurements and neurological status may fit within the 10 abilities. How would you advise them?

Think about a patient you have worked with and apply the Ability Model. Does this case study suggest that there any other factors alongside owner culture, compliance and financial situation that you would advocate adding to the Ability Model?

Consider the clinical focus and the professional values of the team you work with. How would you represent that focus and those values within a model of nursing? Perhaps start by jotting down words to describe the clinical area of focus then add on key priorities and values for care. Share your ideas with a colleague – perhaps you may be able to develop your own practice specific model of care.

References

1. Orpet H and Welsh P (2011). *Handbook of Veterinary Nursing*. Oxford: Wiley Blackwell.
2. Animal Act 2006 [online]. Last accessed 27th March 2017. http://www.legislation .gov.uk/ukpga/2006/45/contents.

Further reading

1. *Culture, Communication and Nursing*. Philip Burnard and Paul Gill (Pearson Education, 2009).

Why should nursing care plans be used in practice?

Chapter 5

Nursing care plans and the patient

By the end of this chapter you will be able to

1. Explain how a nursing care plan may stimulate holistic, patient-centred care within the veterinary environment.
2. Recognise the potential benefits of using nursing care plans to promote continuity of care.
3. Outline the benefits of an effective therapeutic relationship.
4. Explain the communication skills required to support a therapeutic relationship.
5. Describe the application of nursing care plans to the care of chronically ill patients.

Nursing care plans can benefit animals being cared for in veterinary practice in two ways. First, the use of a nursing care plan will facilitate an individualised and thorough assessment which will ensure all the needs of the patient are taken into account. Second, the use of a nursing care plan promotes continuity of care.

Holistic care

The UK Royal College of Veterinary Surgeons code of conduct for veterinary nurses is clear in its assertion that all practicing veterinary nurses are required to put the needs of their patients first, ensuring their priority is always the health and welfare of the animals committed to their care.

By participating in the care planning process, nurses are taking significant steps to fulfil this requirement. A nursing care plan should ensure that all the needs of the patient, their health and their welfare are taken into account. There is evidence that the use of nursing care plans can promote effective patient care. In Brown's [1] case study of an 11-month-old cat who had been involved in a road traffic accident, there was the opportunity to directly compare and contrast care provided with and without a care plan. Brown is clear in her conclusion that comparing the patient's records prior to and following the introduction of a nursing care plan, a more holistic approach was made when a care plan was used. Cited care needs that were addressed after a nursing care plan was put in place included accurate management of calorific requirement through calculation of the recommended energy requirements and the use of gentle massage and grooming to stimulate and soothe the patient. In addition, it was noted that when the nursing care plan was in place, care was spread over the day rather than bunched up in particular parts of the day, which may have left the cat stressed and over stimulated.

Wager and Welsh [2] reinforced these findings in 2013. They observed positive outcomes of using a care model and associated care plan in veterinary nursing, explaining that it supported individualised and patient-specific care. They cite the work of Wager [3] and Lock [4] as additional examples of previously published positive experiences associated with the use of nursing care plans in frontline clinical practice. The evidence is that use of a nursing care plan, implemented as a result of using a structured model of care, can improve care for veterinary patients.

Continuity of care

Alongside the direct benefit of improving patient care, nursing care plans also facilitate continuity of care. A detailed, accurate and contemporary nursing care plan is an invaluable record of the care a patient has received and is due to receive. There are many situations when information about the care of a patient will need to be passed on to a colleague. Patients receiving round the clock care will be cared for by different nurses on different shift patterns. Potentially, the need for specialist care may require the transfer of a patient to a new veterinary hospital. At each of these points a comprehensive transfer of information about the patient must be passed to the new staff. Known colloquially in the medical profession as handover, it has long been known that this passing on of the care of a patient to another colleague is a vulnerable time in terms of patient safety. If handovers are ineffective, clinically relevant information may be omitted or miscommunicated, which in turn may lead to delays in treatment and diagnosis, inappropriate treatment, or even omission of care. The use of a written nursing care plan is an excellent adjuvant to a verbal handover and description of care. In human-centred nursing, community nurses will leave nursing care plans in the homes of their patients, knowing that different nurses may attend and therefore need clear and up-to-date instructions.

Developing a therapeutic relationship

Alongside the explicit benefits of improving patient care and facilitating continuity of care, the use of nursing models and associated nursing care plans have implicit benefits as their use supports the therapeutic relationship between nurse and owner of the animal. Within the context of veterinary nursing, a **therapeutic relationship** may be defined as a series of interactions between a nurse and the owner of an animal that supports effective patient care.

The use of the Orpet and Jeffery Ability Model [5] of care draws the nurse's attention to the importance of the relationship between the owner of the animal and the care that the animal needs and receives. There are two stages in this model. First, there is the emphasis that the model places on obtaining a comprehensive health history from the carer of the animal, which marks the beginning of what hopefully should be a therapeutic relationship between owner and nurse. Second, there is documented emphasis on ensuring that owner compliance is taken into account when planning care.

While comprehensive documentation using a nursing care plan may help multidisciplinary working through improved communication, it is important that in the case of veterinary nursing (much like paediatric human centered nursing) a family-centred approach is advocated. The owner of the animal should be considered an extended member of the multidisciplinary team. There are numerous examples of how a lack of owner adherence to care requirements can directly impact a patient's care, so it is important that a therapeutic relationship is maintained. The clear and concise information found on a nursing care plan may support clear communication and subsequently, support the therapeutic relationship between nurse and owner.

A key advantage of developing a therapeutic relationship with an owner or carer of an animal is that the veterinary nurse may get to know the owner better and design a care plan that takes into account the owner's needs. There is no point in writing out clear discharge instructions for an owner who struggles to read. While illiteracy is rarely something that people admit openly, there may be tell-tale signs noticed as a veterinary nurse spends time with an owner. This may lead to a modification of the approach to an owner, so less reliance on written materials and more on diagrams or practical demonstrations. A further example is when veterinary nurses are caring for animals owned by healthcare professionals, discharging a newly diabetic cat to a diabetic nurse specialist will likely need a different approach than discharging to someone who doesn't know what diabetes is. Assumptions of their knowledge should never be made, but it is likely they will have a higher level of understanding generally.

A therapeutic relationship will allow a nurse to openly consider the other factors advocated for consideration within Orpet and Jeffery's Ability Model, including the culture of the owner and the financial situation of the owner. Being able to have open and frank conversations about such things should enable the team to make adaptations to care to support the owner and therefore provide better care to the animal. Through such relationships patient-centred plans of care may be made. With diligent owner education and support, care that has traditionally been reserved to a veterinary hospital environment may be moved in the home. There are multiple benefits to being able to facilitate this; the animal is likely to suffer less stress, feeling more comfortable in their own environment. The owner may reduce both their trips to the vets and the financial impact of the animal's treatment by providing care at home. A prime example is addressing nutritional needs when owners of animals may be taught to administer enteral nutrition, just as human-centred nurses will teach their patients to manage their own feeding regimen through gastrostomy tubes.

Communication and the therapeutic relationship

Empathy and compassion are key characteristics of a positive therapeutic relationship. To communicate effectively, nurses must demonstrate empathy and compassion. Difficult to define due to the subjective nature of both, and potentially more difficult to identify, empathy is considered the ability to consider the situation or circumstances of another person without acknowledging personal feelings on the matter. Compassion is a reflection of the relationship between the nurse and patient, or in the case of veterinary nursing, also between the nurse and animal's owner. It should incorporate kindness and the recognition of suffering and vulnerability. Being able to demonstrate compassion and empathy are the foundations of a therapeutic relationship, if both are present owners are more likely to trust nurses, confide in them and therefore work with them to promote the health of their animal. Nurses should concentrate on developing skills to listen actively to ensure that they understand and clarify what owners may be saying to them. They should also ensure they work collaboratively, with both the owner and their colleagues to ensure that information provided is accurate and relevant.

One of the key barriers to a therapeutic relationship is when healthcare teams make assumptions. A nurse may write the most detailed home-care plan, full of useful hints and tips for caring for the pet with advice and guidance. However, if initial conversations have not taken place and the veterinary team have simply assumed that the owner will be able to manage, afford and facilitate the required care, when in fact the owner cannot, it is likely to mark a negative start to the long-term care of the animal.

When trying to develop effective relationships with owners, nurses need to be mindful of their own thoughts, emotions and feelings. **Emotional intelligence** is often discussed in the context of those working in the caring professions. It is associated with an ability to recognise, express, and, possibly most importantly, control one's own emotions. Nursing patients with long term conditions can be difficult emotionally. Owners are ultimately the decision makers and it might be hard for nurses to facilitate decisions that they perceive to be wrong or misguided. Nurses need to pay attention to their emotional intelligence and take steps to promote it through consideration of coping strategies such as establishing a sensible work-life balance, taking regular time off, spending time with family and friends and potentially using reflective practice to address any concerns and move forward.

Furthermore, it can be very difficult to display compassion for others when nurses are not working within a compassionate environment and not being treated with compassion themselves. A mutual respect for colleagues despite personal differences may be difficult to sustain, but will contribute towards better outcomes for patients and their owners.

Self-care plans in human-centred nursing

There are several areas of care within human-centred nursing where patients are encouraged to think ahead and make their own care plans in discussion with their friends and family.

If patients are to be encouraged to read and agree to plans of care, conversation must be open so that the patient understands their own medical situation. It is the patient's right to know what their care plan entails. It is likely that in knowing and understanding what the plan is, they are far more likely to comply and achieve the goal associated with the planned intervention.

Patients with chronic disease may well become experts in managing their symptoms. They will use the relevant drugs appropriately and liaise with various members of their multidisciplinary team as required. Self-care plans will often lay out strategies for step up therapies for exacerbations of their condition alongside instructions for daily care and medication.

A nursing care plan written with the patient that the patient can take home with them can guide the patient's self-care when staying at home. Managing and treating early symptoms may well be safer than leaving them until the patient is weak, unwell, admitted to hospital, and consequently, more at risk from infection through being recumbent with a compromised immune status.

An excellent example of a patient's self-care plan that is used regularly is the lung self-care plan, used in the author's workplace, Papworth Hospital NHS Foundation Trust. The Lung Defence Unit is a team of healthcare professionals who look after patients with difficult lung infections. The case mix includes patients suffering from primary and secondary immunodeficiency syndromes, aspergillus-related lung disease, rheumatoid arthritis, serious childhood infection and chronic aspiration. The self-care plan provides a comprehensive resource for patients to use to manage their condition in partnership with the multidisciplinary team (Figure 5.1).

Palliative care within the NHS is used in chronic disease. Palliative care teams are experts at controlling the symptoms that accompany the end stages of chronic disease. They develop care plans that view the patient as a whole, administering synergistic medication that can provide relief of a variety of symptoms. Furthermore, they will plan those interventions with the patient. Different people will prioritise different symptoms to deal with and only the patient can decide how they want their symptoms managed. A medication review might be indicated and yet again, patient involvement is key. Patients may potentially opt to discontinue some of their treatment medication to eliminate unpleasant side effects.

Some people wish to spend their last weeks and months at home, some feel more comfortable in hospital. These discussions are had in advance and plans put in place with the agreement of

My rescue treatments

♦ **Antibiotics**
♦ **Steroids**

Discuss keeping a rescue pack at home with your GP
Other advice for exacerbations:

You should contact the Lung Defence Telephone Support Service if
- **your symptoms worsen despite taking your rescue treatments**
- **you need your rescue treatments more than 3 times a year**

My follow up
My follow up will be by telephone / in clinic

You should have a list of your current medications, a record of any chest infections since your last review and any questions you may want to ask to hand.

Useful Resources

My self management plan

Name:

Hospital Number:

My Allergies:

My normal daily symptoms

Sputum volume:

Sputum colour:

Sputum thickness:

I cough:

Exercise: I can usually:

Figure 5.1 Self-care plan for people with chronic lung disease. (Reproduced from Papworth Hospital NHS Foundation Trust. With kind permission.)

the patient. These plans are then documented and shared with the multidisciplinary team and family members.

Patients holding their own care plans is not particularly novel. Care plans for the under-fives have been held at their home with their parents for many years. The 'red book' has documented nursing care, provided healthcare goals, guidelines and care notes, and is often a regularly used document of care. People are familiar with this model and it is a huge source of information and a useful tool for continuity of care.

Currently, it may be assumed that most veterinary treatment of animals in the UK occurs within a veterinary environment. Even though nursing care plans are more likely to be used in the veterinary environment, is there any reason why their use cannot be extended to the home environment as well? Owners very often extend veterinary care through the administration of regular medication, monitoring and specific feeding after education and training from the veterinary team.

A prime example of the extension of the veterinary care of animals is the care owners provide after a patient has undergone a routine elective procedure. These procedures, such as neutering are completed as day cases, under general anaesthesia. When owners arrive to collect their animal and take them home, they are often given very specific instructions regarding home care, including management of medication, diet and exercise. Knowing that when owners collect their animal they are very often distracted and unable to concentrate on the information from the vet or nurse, written instructions are often provided. These support the verbal information exchange and many veterinary teams have been providing such information sheets for years. These standardised care sheets are, essentially, nursing care plans, specific instructions designed to facilitate care of the animal at home (Figure 5.2).

Care planning and chronic illness

The care planning process is very often applied to animals who are acutely ill inpatients at the veterinary hospital. However, if the evidence demonstrates that using the care planning process and the associated care plans may improve the care of veterinary patients, might the same process equally be applied to outpatients who are chronically ill?

A chronic condition of ill health may be defined as one that continues for a long period, or recurs regularly over time. In the context of veterinary nursing, chronic health conditions in animals also have the added characteristic that they require care input from their owners.

Consideration of chronic ill health in animals must go hand in hand with consideration of quality of life. Quality of life is a complex subject, and the subject of much debate within human-centred nursing. Numerous definitions and tools are available to try and measure quality of life. Ultimately many of them are designed so that the impact of the care of chronic health conditions might be measured. Assessing quality of life is equally complex in animals, and often relies on a subjective assessment between the veterinary team and the owner, taking into consideration factors such as ability to exercise, pain levels, perceived enjoyment of activities, and ability to perform normal bodily functions such as toileting, eating, and drinking.

Owners who are caring for animals who are chronically ill benefit from a therapeutic relationship with veterinary nurses. Many veterinary nurses have evolved their role to include the assessment, monitoring, and support of chronically ill outpatients. The development of such a role may be due to a combination of logistics and communication skills. Some veterinary nurses simply have more flexibility in planning their day to facilitate accessible clinical appointments to discuss chronic health conditions in detail and assist owners to understand the care their pet needs. Some veterinary nurses may possess better communication skills than their veterinary surgeon colleagues and consequently, owners may prefer speaking with a veterinary nurse and may confide more to a nurse than a vet, allowing the nurse to develop a more specific care plan.

Chronically ill animals require regular assessment, in combination with discussions surrounding quality of life. Through these regular assessments and therapeutic interactions with the veterinary team, therapy may be optimised, often through a combination of nursing interventions. The support of these owners and their animals also requires a forward-thinking approach so that future appointments may be booked and new interventions followed up to ensure that owners are happy and able to administrate the care required.

Aims of supporting an owner to care for a chronically ill animal at home

1. Optimise the health and welfare of the animal.
2. Provide the best possible patient experience for animal and owner.

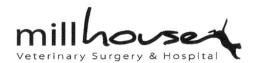

Veterinary Surgery & Hospital

20 Tennyson Avenue • Kings Lynn • Norfolk • PE30 2QG • www.millhouse vets.co.uk
Telephone: 01553 771457 • Fax: 01553 761115 • email: admin@millhousevets. co.uk • Vat No: 115 1416 58

YOUR PET'S RECOVERY AFTER SURGERY

VET Solutions   06.03.2017
25 The Street
Kings Lynn
Kings Lynn

Please read these notes carefully.

Poochie has undergone surgery for which a sedative or general anaesthetic was given, and will probably be sleepy for at least 24 hours as the effects of the anaesthetic or sedative wear off. You may see a small shaved area on one front leg where the anaesthetic or sedative was administered. If blood samples have been taken there may be a shaved area under the neck. The hair will soon grow back.

Please encourage Poochie to eat the food provided. We would recommend that you feed this up to the time of the post operative check, when we will discuss long term feeding of your pet - purchase more supplies at reception. Allow Poochie free access to water at all times. Follow the instructions of the veterinary surgeon or veterinary nurse regarding exercise and long term feeding.

It is vitally important to stop Poochie from licking and chewing at the wound and surrounding area, as this delays healing and can introduce infection into the surgical wound. If this seems impossible, or the area looks red, sore or is uncomfortable, please contact the surgery straight away. If, during the convalescent period, you are worried in any way about Poochie, please do not hesitate to telephone the surgery where one of the veterinary nurses or veterinary surgeons will be only too happy to discuss your concerns.

Poochie 's next check up is due: , with:

Treatments to be given:

_____ RVN

The nurse that has discharged Poochie today is _____
Today they have given you advice regarding:
☐ Feeding Poochie post-operatively and future dietary requirements
   Poochie 's weight today is 1.00 kg. The Body Fat Index is   %, ie.   risk.
☐ Wound care, bandage protection and the use of protection collars (available to buy at reception)
☐ Exercise and any special requirements that the vet has requested whilst Poochie is recovering

---

Figure 5.2 In practice – Post-operative information sheet for owners. (Reproduced from Mill House Veterinary Hospital. With kind permission.)

(*Continued*)

Post – Neutering Timetable

1st Post Op Check – at 2 days (not usually needed for cat castrates) to check your cat is recovering well after surgery	Date .... Time ....
2nd Post Op Check – at 10 days to check that recovery is progressing as expected	Date .... Time ....
1st Weight Check – after 3 months To make sure your cat is progressing well in the longer term and to check whether your cat's weight is fluctuating – we can advise you on the best diet for them.	Date .... Time .... Recorded weight ....kg Recommendations ....
2nd Weight Check – after 6 months	Date .... Time .... Recorded weight ....kg Recommendations ....

millhouse   20 Tennyson Avenue Kings Lynn Norfolk PE30 2QG t: +44 (0)1553 771457 e: info@millhousevets.co.uk w: www.millhousevets.co.uk RCVS

After Your Cat is Neutered

Today .... has been neutered.

Treatments to be given ....

Additional Advice...

....

The nurse that has discharged .... today is ....

They have given you advice regarding:
- Post-operative feeding and future dietary requirements
- Wound care, bandage protection and the use of protection collars (available to buy at reception)
- Exercise and any special requirements that the vet has requested while your pet is recovering

This leaflet covers:
- Post-op care
- Preventing interference with the wound
- The right nutrition for your neutered cat
- Aftercare timetable

Today your cat has been neutered. The operation is not reversible, and a neutered cat will never be able to breed. If your cat is female, she has been spayed (a full ovariohysterectomy – the womb and ovaries have been removed) in which case she will have a shaved area and stitches (which may be dissolvable and within the skin) on her left side. If your cat is male he has been castrated (both testicles have been removed through the scrotum) –

no stitches are needed. Both will have a small shaved area on the front leg where we gave the anaesthetic. If blood samples have been taken there may be a shaved area under the neck. The hair usually takes several weeks to grow back.

How long does it take for my cat to recover?

Usually, cats are able to go home the same day, and recover well, although female cats are quieter than males as they have had a more complex operation. Your pet may be sleepy for at least 24 hours as the effects of the anaesthetic wears off. Feeding an easy to digest diet is important and you have been offered a special diet that is easy to eat, gentle on the stomach and high in nutrients to aid recovery. You should feed this for several days. We advise keeping all cats indoors for 10 days until they are fully recovered, and you will need to make an appointment for spayed females to come back in 2 days for a check up, and in 10 days to have any stitches removed.

Male cats need a check up after a week to ensure everything is well. At this time most cats are back to normal. The check up appointments are generally with a nurse, and there is no charge for these.

millhouse   20 Tennyson Avenue Kings Lynn Norfolk PE30 2QG t: +44 (0)1553 771457 e: info@millhousevets.co.uk w: www.millhousevets.co.uk RCVS

Keeping your cat comfortable after the operation

Your cat has been given pain relief, which should last between 36 and 48 hours but please help us by looking for the following signs which may indicate that more treatment is needed:
- Withdrawn or quiet
- Trembling, or pacing
- Crying out
- Aggressive behaviour when handled, or guarding the painful area
- Biting or licking at the painful area
- Increased heart rate, panting, dilated pupils, increased temperature
- Not eating

Cats in pain may show only one or two of these signs, or may just be a little quieter than usual. If you are unsure how to recognise these signs, or you think your cat is in pain, please telephone us for advice or come to the surgery.

Pain Relief

We use Non-Steroidal Anti- Inflammatory Drugs (NSAIDs), given as tablets or liquids, for example **Metacam** (meloxicam) to keep your cat comfortable. NSAID's must be given WITH FOOD to avoid stomach upsets and stomach ulcers.

Always follow dosage instructions carefully and consult us if you feel the drugs are not working, or you wish to reduce the dose.

> **Cats handle drugs differently to people, so <u>never</u> use human drugs for them without veterinary instructions. In particular, aspirin and paracetomol are very toxic to cats.**

How to protect the wound

It is often said that licking can encourage healing – but this is absolutely not so - licking introduces infection into an area and does not encourage healing.

Unfortunately, we cannot explain this to a cat, nor prevent interference sufficiently by just watching and distracting

our patients when they lick. A protection collar or a medical pet shirt can allow your cat's wound to heal properly and more quickly without disruption from your cat.

> **We may not offer you a petshirt or collar for your cat if he/she seems relaxed and unlikely to lick or interfere with the operation site. Please ask for one, however, if you see any sign of licking or if your cat has done this before.**

General Recommendations

Please follow our instructions regarding your cat's activity during the recovery period.

Observe the wound, surgical site, or dressings – please report to us any swelling, discharge or smell.

Feed the special recovery food, Hill's feline i/d. It will aid your cat's recovery, as well as supporting their digestive health. This is always available for purchase from reception.

If you have another pet in the house, make sure that they do not lick or interfere with the wound.

millhouse   20 Tennyson Avenue Kings Lynn Norfolk PE30 2QG t: +44 (0)1553 771457 e: info@millhousevets.co.uk w: www.millhousevets.co.uk RCVS

If you have any concerns about your cat's recovery at any time please contact the surgery and we will be happy to help.

If a protection collar is used

We will fit the protection collar correctly for you so that your cat cannot remove it.

Your cat may react negatively to the collar at first, but they will usually learn to accept it within 24 hours. If your cat is still upset by the collar after this time please contact us for advice.

Your cat will usually be able to sleep, eat and drink with the collar on.

Please do not be tempted to remove the collar without our advise – a cat can destroy their wound within minutes.

Check your cat's neck and ears for signs of irritation and contact us if you notice anything unusual.

Keep the collar clean by washing with soap and water.

It is particularly important for your cat to wear the collar when unsupervised and overnight.

Do I have to do anything differently after neutering?

Feed nutrition specifically formulated for neutered cats to keep your cat fit

Neutered cats may look the same but they need different nutrition to avoid health problems, such as gaining excess weight.
We strongly recommend starting your cat on **Hill's Lower Fat VetEssentials Neutered Cat** right after neutering. This advanced nutrition with clinically proven health benefits is specifically formulated to meet the essential health needs of neutered cats. It contains appropriate levels of protein and fat to help maintain your cat's ideal weight as well as controlled mineral and pH levels to maintain healthy urinary tract. Ask us about special offers and vouchers for Vetessentials. Your pet likes it or we buy it back!

It is estimated that one in four cats in Europe are overweight – make sure your cat eats well and stays trim. Our Veterinary Health Advisors are all fully qualified nurses and will be able to help – **consultations and regular weighing are free.**

Weigh your cat regularly to ensure they are not gaining weight after neutering

We recommend a weight check after 3 months and again after 6 months.

Don't forget to ensure your cat's microchip is regularly scanned and to keep up with annual vaccination, flea and worming preventative treatments and health examinations.

Any queries?
Don't hesitate to phone on
01553 771457

millhouse   20 Tennyson Avenue Kings Lynn Norfolk PE30 2QG t: +44 (0)1553 771457 e: info@millhousevets.co.uk w: www.millhousevets.co.uk RCVS

Figure 5.2 (*Continued*) In practice – Post-operative information sheet for owners. (Reproduced from Mill House Veterinary Hospital. With kind permission.)

There are two aims of supporting an owner to care for their chronically ill animal at home. The primary aim must always be to promote the health of the animal and achieve positive clinical outcomes, the relief of pain for example, or optimal blood glucose control. A secondary aim is to provide a better patient experience, for both owner and animal. Therapeutic relationships built up over time facilitate care of both owner and animal that is specific to them. It allows the veterinary nurse to think laterally and provide care that might not be routine, but suits a particular set of circumstances. Follow up appointments might be booked several weeks or months ahead to fit into work patterns. Advice and support might be provided by phone and email, rather than relying exclusively on face to face consultations. Home visits might suit other owners and allow assistance to be provided with medication or monitoring of a patient's condition.

Home-care plans

In her 2016 article, Belinda Marchbank discussed the idea of extending the use of nursing theory, the nursing process, nursing models and nursing care plans to chronically ill patients living at home. One of the biggest challenges in supporting owners to care for chronically ill animals is knowing what information is relevant and what the best possible way of giving that information to an owner might be. The use of the veterinary nursing process, in combination with a model of care, may produce a care plan which a nurse and owner may use together to facilitate home care.

Marchbank's chronic illness management plan (CHIMP) was designed to use the same parameters as that of the Ability Model from Orpet and Jeffery. Like the self-care plans used in human-centred nursing, it provides a template whereby the veterinary nurse may assess the needs of the patient and create a written record of the nursing interventions the owner can carry out at home to support the health and wellbeing of their animal. Perhaps, given the reliance most animals have on their owners, adapting the title, self-care plan, used most often in human-centred nursing, to home-care plan, is more appropriate for the veterinary nursing profession. Using the CHIMP model, a home-care plan may provide details of the medication the patient requires, with space to include the particulars of future planned appointments, explanation of the diagnosis, and details of any potential complications of the diagnosis (Figure 5.3) [6].

Borrowing from and adapting the self-care plans from human-centred nursing, veterinary home-care plans may also include details of resources owners can use to further their understanding of the condition of their animal. As previously discussed, health literacy in the UK is rising, the general public are much more likely to know and understand their own health condition having used resources from the Internet. This may account for the rising number of animal owners keen to learn more about their pet's health and welfare from internet sites or other owners in the same situation. Taking the time to construct a list of useful, relevant resources that owners might use to further their understanding may prevent confusion and worry that can be caused by undirected web browsing. Common misconceptions include the direct application of human-centred medicine to veterinary patients, or confusion surrounding the use of human drugs for animal patients, so particular instructions might be provided, for example, do not use paracetamol. Additionally, as with human-centred self-care plans, the inclusion of the contact details of who should be called should the animals condition deteriorate is useful.

Such home-care plans are useful tools in supporting patient care in the home environment. The advantages of using such a care plan in chronic illness echo the advantages of using a nursing care plan in practice for inpatients. There are advantages to both the patients and the nursing team responsible for the animal's care.

Education

Patient name: ....Date: ....

Client name: ....

Diagnosis: ....

Explanation of disease: ....
....
....
....

The client will need to know the name of the disease their pet has been diagnosed with. They will also need an explanation of the disease process and how the disease will affect their pet.

Medications:

Name	Dose	Duration	Special instructions

Each medication that the pet requires should be listed out here. Special instructions could include use gloves, store in fridge, give 1 hour before food, etc.

Ongoing monitoring and care

Revisit schedule

Date	Length	Purpose	Estimated Cost

It is important to set the clients up for success. Giving them the details of the revisits such as how often, what will be done at each revisit and the approximate cost will allow them to plan for these and increase compliance which will ultimately result in better outcomes for the animal.

Diet: ....
....

Prescription diets can form part of the management and/or treatment of many diseases. It is important that the clients are clear about the diet required, how it benefits and how to transition to this diet from the pet's current diet.

Water: ....
....
....

The water requirements or thirst of the patient can be impacted significantly by either the disease itself or by the medication required to treat the disease. Clients will need clear advice about whether to provide extra water dishes or how to monitor the water intake of their pet.

Toileting: ....
....

The water and food intake can in turn influence the toileting behaviour of the animal. Clients need clear advice about this; they may need to increase the frequency of toilet stops for their pet.

Mobility: ....
....

Activity and rest: ....
....

Mobility and hence the activity and rest requirements of the patient can be impacted by either the disease itself or by the treatment.

Clients will need advice about whether to: increase/decrease activity, provide physiotherapy, change the type of exercise the animal is doing, etc.

Behaviour: ....
....

Disease often has a significant impact on an animal's behaviour.

The client will need to know what changes to expect from the disease or from the treatment.

Potential complications: ....
....

Symptoms can change and new ones can develop as a disease progresses.

It is important that the client knows what to look for so that they can monitor their pet's progress and return to the clinic when appropriate.

Notes: ....
....
....
....
....

If you are ever concerned about your pet please call the clinic immediately.

Figure 1. The Chronic Illness Management Plan.

Figure 5.3 Chronic illness management plan (CHIMP). (Reproduced from Marchbank B, *The Veterinary Nurse*, 7, 312, 2016. With permission from The Veterinary Nurse Editor.)

Things to include in a home-care plan for chronically ill animals

- Patient identification details
- Diagnosis
- Explanation of diagnosis
- Medications – including dose, duration of use and any specific instructions for use
- Details of follow up appointments, at the practice, via email or telephone
- Contact details of veterinary team caring for the animal
- Nursing interventions according to the CHIMP model (diet, water, toileting, mobility, activity and rest and behaviour)
- Details of any potential complications and their associated signs and symptoms
- Details of useful resources for further reading and comprehension of the condition
- Space for notes so owners may jot down comments or questions

The home-care plan will facilitate holistic, individualised care; it will ensure that all the needs of the patient are addressed. It provides a record of the nursing care and the information given to the owner, fulfilling professional requirements surrounding record keeping. Additionally, copies of the home-care plan may be made so that any other people who will be responsible for the animal will have clear and concise instructions. This is useful for animals that may need to go into a kennel or cattery, or spend time in doggy day-care, or with pet-sitters when owners are away or at work (Figure 5.4).

Discussing complex chronic conditions can be challenging, the aim is to support the owner to comprehend and ultimately manage their animal's health in conjunction with the veterinary team. Yet again, the owner becomes part of the multidisciplinary team. The home-care plan may be used as a communication tool for the veterinary team, providing a structure to the nurse – owner interaction, as it is filled in, step by step. Clear and concise communication is the cornerstone of all therapeutic relationships. While the written home-care plan may support and reinforce the process, it shouldn't be used as a complete substitute for discussion and explanation.

HOME CARE PLAN

PATIENT NAME   Lionel

CLIENT NAME   Ballantyne lane

DIAGNOSIS   Feline lower urinary tract disease (FLUTD)

EXPLANATION   FLUTD is not a specific disease, but actually a term that covers the symptoms Lionel has experienced, straining to urinate, pain on urination and urinary blockage

MEDICATIONS NAME	DOSE		DURATION	SPECIAL INSTRUCTIONS
BUPRENORPHINE	0.2 mL	three x daily under the tongue	For 2 days	
MELOXICAM	dose for 3 kg	with food once daily	For 5 days	Monitor for signs of vomiting or diarrhoea
PRAZOSIN	0.5 mg	orally twice daily	Complete course	

VETERINARY APPOINTMENTS DATE	TIME	PURPOSE	COST

No further check ups planned unless you are concerned that Lionel is having problems urinating

DIET	Please feed a wet diet twice daily this will ↑ Lionel's water intake
WATER	Encourage Lionel to drink regularly, consider use of cat fountain or adding water to his meals
TOILETING	Monitor Lionel's urination closely, contact us if you have any concerns
MOBILITY	Lionel can have free access to house + garden as before his illness
ACTIVITY + REST	Lionel is unrestricted in activity + rest
BEHAVIOUR	Please monitor Lionel's behaviour, changes to his usual behaviour or routine such as urinating in inappropriate places may indicate he has cystitis again
POTENTIAL COMPLICATIONS	
NOTES	Thank you for the insurance claim form, will submit it on your behalf in next 14 days

If you would like to read more about Lionel's conditions, details can be found at www.goodinfoaboutyourpet.com

Figure 5.4 **In practice – Home-care plan. (Adapted from Marchbank B,** *The Veterinary Nurse,* **7, 312, 2016. With permission from The Veterinary Nurse Editor.)**

Review

- Nursing care plans can improve patient care for animals admitted to veterinary care. Additionally, nursing care plans support individualised care which can promote patient health and wellbeing.
- Therapeutic relationships with the owners of patients rely on the demonstration of empathy, compassion and emotional intelligence.
- Continuity of care is an important factor in keeping patients safe; nursing care plans are a valuable tool to support continuity of care.
- Nursing care plans may also be applied to chronically ill patients living at home, supporting their health and providing a more positive patient experience with the veterinary team.

Future reflections

Consider some of the surgical and medical interventions that are frequently carried out within your practice. Do you provide home-care plans for the owners of patients who have undergone those procedures? Now consider the procedures that are less frequently carried out. Does your practice also have home-care plans for those patients having those procedures too? If not, consider designing and writing some. Do you think it is more important to have home-care plans for patients undergoing routine elective surgery, or for patients that are undergoing surgical or medical interventions that are not carried out frequently at your practice? Why might the owners of animals who are undergoing more unusual treatments benefit more from detailed home-care plans?

References

1. Brown C (`2012). Experience of designing and implementing a care plan in the veterinary environment. *The Veterinary Nurse*, 3 (9), 534–542.
2. Welsh P and Wager C (2013). Veterinary nurses creating a unique approach to patient care: Part one. *The Veterinary Nurse*, 4 (8), 452–459.
3. Wager C (2011). Case study: A critical reflection of implementing a nursing care plan for two hospitalised patients. *The Veterinary Nurse*, 2 (6), 328–332.
4. Lock K (2011). Reflections on designing and implementing a nursing care plan. *The Veterinary Nurse*, 2 (5), 272–277.
5. Orpet H and Welsh P (2011). *Handbook of Veterinary Nursing*. 2nd ed. Oxford: Wiley-Blackwell.
6. Marchbank B (2016). The chronic illness management plan. *The Veterinary Nurse*, 7 (6), 310–317.

Further reading

There is a large amount of human-centred resources about communication skills that may be adapted to use within the veterinary profession to support effective therapeutic relationships between veterinary nurse and owner.

1. *Compassion, Caring and Communication Skills for Nursing Practice*. Jacqui Baughan and Ann Smith (Pearson, 2013).
2. *Communication and Interpersonal Skills for Nurses*. Shirley Bach and Alec Grant (Learning Matters, 2009).
3. *Interpersonal Relationships – Professional Communication Skills for Nurses*, 7th edition. Elizabeth C Arnold and Kathleen Underman Boggs (Elsevier, 2016).

Chapter 6

Nursing care plans and the professional veterinary nurse

By the end of this chapter you will be able to

1. Describe the characteristics of a profession.
2. Explain how the use of nursing care plans may support professionalism within veterinary nursing.
3. Outline how nursing care plans may facilitate effective multidisciplinary teamworking.
4. Recognise the principles of advocacy and how nursing care plans may support nurses to be advocates for their patients.
5. Debate the impact of the use of nursing theory, models and care plans on the role of the veterinary nurse within the veterinary team and wider society.

Defining a profession

The idea that the use of veterinary nursing care plans may support veterinary nursing in establishing itself as a profession is a complex concept. Defining the characteristics of a profession is a subject that has been much debated over the years. The most basic definition of a profession is a role or occupation that requires the learning of specific knowledge and requires members to adhere to a code of conduct.

Key characteristics of a profession

1. Having a specific body of knowledge
2. Working to a code of conduct

In 2015, all listed veterinary nurses in the UK, those who had completed Royal College of Veterinary Surgeons accredited training in veterinary nursing, became registered veterinary nurses. As a result, they committed to working to a code of conduct which directs both their professional and personal conduct. With this change, veterinary nursing in the UK took giant steps towards becoming a profession in its own right, able to demonstrate that it was beginning to fulfil the generally accepted characteristics of a profession.

The concept that veterinary nursing has its own specific knowledge is probably the most difficult characteristic for the profession to demonstrate. Defining veterinary nursing knowledge is not easy. There is so much that may be medical, physiological and biological information and therefore shared with other professions such as veterinary surgeons, doctors, dentists and midwives.

There is one clear defining characteristic of veterinary nursing that sets it apart from the other related professions. That characteristic is the requirement of VNs to take into account the needs of the whole patient, to provide holistic care.

The application and consideration of the veterinary nursing process, models of nursing care, and associated nursing care plans all support holistic care, which ensures all the needs of the patient are considered. Therefore, through the use of such tools, it may be demonstrated that veterinary nursing is beginning to build its own specific body of knowledge unique to the veterinary nursing profession.

Establishing a code of conduct for veterinary nurses was a key step in establishing veterinary nursing as a profession. Using nursing care plans can support veterinary nurses to fulfil their professional responsibilities in adhering to the code of conduct. In the UK, collaborative working within the multidisciplinary team, record-keeping, professional accountability and ensuring VNs provide adequate and appropriate care are all mandated by the RCVS Code of Conduct. Each of these concepts may be supported through the use of nursing care plans. In fact it might be argued that the nursing care plan is the single most useful tool VNs have at their disposal to fulfil the requirements of the UK code of conduct.

Alongside the explicit professional benefits of nursing care plans, supporting veterinary nursing specific knowledge and assisting veterinary nurses to adhere to the code of conduct, there are also more subtle, implicit benefits which may arise. It might be speculated that the use of a nursing care plan by nurses who are supporting owners looking after chronically ill animals at home may well raise the awareness of the role of the veterinary nurse with the general public.

Additionally, veterinary nursing care plans may increase the morale and professional satisfaction levels of veterinary nurses. They may empower VNs to advocate for their patients when care needs are omitted or neglected, which may promote professional satisfaction as nurses help provide the very best care for an animal. Finally, the use of nursing care plans may also help VNs contribute to the commercial nature of the veterinary business.

Professional benefits of using nursing care plans

1. Thorough documentation of clinical decision-making to support accountability
2. Improved multidisciplinary teamworking
3. Increased professional satisfaction for veterinary nurses
4. Improved public perception of the role of the veterinary nurse
5. Increased revenue for veterinary practice

Nursing care plans and professional accountability

A contemporary, comprehensive nursing care plan may provide an excellent record of care. Such records will be adjusted and adapted as the care is given, and can also be referred to retrospectively should clinical decisions be challenged. Historically, documentation of nursing care was completed for therapeutic reasons. It facilitated continuity of care and assisted with care planning. Now, documentation has an additional purpose: it can support professional accountability. Veterinary nurses are personally accountable for their professional practice and they must be able to justify their decisions and actions.

Using a nursing model in combination with the veterinary nursing process to produce a care plan will enable nurses to justify the care they have given throughout the treatment journey of the patient. They will be able to demonstrate that they have a thorough understanding of their patient's needs, having completed a holistic assessment. Should there be an unexpected poor outcome for a patient while it is under veterinary care, nursing documentation may be scrutinised so that the outcome may be understood and potentially prevented in the future. Detailed documentation is the best protection that a nurse can have if they find themselves involved in a complaint or grievance surrounding an animal they have nursed. No matter how poignant the case was, or how recent, it will still be difficult to recall all the details of the care without clear contemporary records. Equally important, records of care for patients who thrived under veterinary care may be examined. They can be used as education tools, to share knowledge and good practice.

The concept of professional accountability may be daunting to members of such a young profession as veterinary nursing. However, a sensible nurse will always document care carefully and effectively, for therapeutic reasons, with the needs of the patient in mind, rather than to support accountability. In doing so, they will undoubtedly be creating robust documentation that will withstand any examination.

Nursing care plans and multidisciplinary team working

Nursing care plans may be a useful tool to support multidisciplinary communication. Clear communication and collaborative working is a positive characteristic of most professions. In the UK it is mandated by the veterinary nurse's code of conduct. The RCVS advises that VNs must communicate with their colleagues to ensure the health and welfare of their patients.

The process of care planning encourages the development of goals of care. Sharing such goals of care among team members may contribute to greater team cohesion, the ability to plan workloads, and potentially, a happier working environment. In addition, taking the time to ensure all members of a patient's healthcare team understand and agree with the care goals supports clear lines of communication with the patient or patient's owner.

Multidisciplinary team meetings are common within medical healthcare where joint decisions may be made using the input of several professional groups. Members of the multidisciplinary team may include doctors from surgery, medicine and radiology; nurses, including specialist nurses; physiotherapists; dieticians; occupational therapists; psychologists; psychiatrists and social workers. A common scenario at such meetings are discussions surrounding discharge planning. Consider a patient who has had complex heart surgery with a week-long stay on the intensive care unit. While the surgeon might be happy that the procedure has been carried out with good effect and feels secure that the heart is functioning well, other members of the team may have different concerns. Even short periods on intensive care can cause a loss of physical function through muscle wastage and critical care neuropathy. Physiotherapy is an important part of recovery, and rehabilitation back to an appropriate level of function is essential before a patient may be discharged. Therefore, while the doctor may hold seniority in qualification and experience, they will respect the input of the physiotherapist who asks for another two days to work alongside the occupational health team in ensuring that the patient has all the assistance they require at home to facilitate their care and continued rehabilitation. It is also important to ensure that the patient is consulted and agrees with any goals of care that are set. Without their agreement, it can be very difficult to move forward with care.

While sharing agreed care goals is common between veterinary nurses and veterinary surgeons, it may be less common for those goals to be shared with other members of the veterinary multidisciplinary team, the administrative staff, practice managers, nursing care assistants, or receptionists. There are clear advantages in sharing such information with these members of the team.

It is important to remember that each member of staff will have their own unique role in a patient's care. While veterinary nurses and veterinary surgeons have been giving direct veterinary care, the nursing care assistant may have been responsible for supporting the veterinary nursing team and, therefore, the patient. For example, they may have instigated barrier nursing for a patient during their stay ensuring that personal protective equipment is available and appropriate cleaning guidelines are adhered to. The administrative team in the practice office may have been working with the owner's insurance company to support the financial settlement of the care. The receptionists may get to know owners of animals undergoing regular or longer term stays at the hospital as they come and visit and may therefore be in a prime position to offer some support and understanding.

Keeping all the members of the multidisciplinary team up to date may help each team member plan their work. So, if a complex case that has been hospitalised for several days needs further diagnostics and imaging, this will have a direct impact on the financial outcome of the care. The practice manager may benefit from knowing this information as soon as possible to allow them to direct their work. They may contact the owner to ensure they know estimates have changed, or speak to a patient's insurance company. The receptionist, who knows that the owners are due to come in at 2 pm, would benefit from knowing that there are plans to perform imaging and that it might be difficult for owners to visit at that time. They may be able to intercept the owners and reorganise their visiting time, or at least explain why they cannot visit at the time planned when they arrive.

Furthermore, imagine that same patient takes a turn for the worse. Again, it is important that key staff are kept aware. The nursing assistant needs to know so they are not trying to encourage the dog to walk when they are uncomfortable. The receptionist needs to know that the owners are coming in to potentially hear the worst news and therefore be prepared to offer them appropriate support. The management team might benefit from knowing so they can plan their work accordingly. Members of the management or administration team may have worked with owners to develop payment plans, or complete insurance claim forms. If staff are not aware the patient's condition has changed, they may inadvertently offend the owners by trying to address complex financial arrangements at the same time they are being told their pet might not survive. It would obviously not be the best time to discuss such issues.

In most veterinary practices, keeping everyone up to date about every case every day is probably not necessary nor particularly easy to facilitate. Client confidentiality also applies and information should only be shared on a need-to-know basis. Most practices will do a ward round or handover and, at this point, relevant personnel may be invited. Alternatively, members of the team at the meeting may be given the responsibility of ensuring other staff are aware of plans for care and therefore able to contribute as required. Using a nursing care plan to record the care needs and goals is an ideal solution as the information is available for all to access should they need it. All team members should be trained as to the function and format of the care plan so they are able to pick out the information most relevant to them.

Nursing care plans and professional satisfaction

A care plan, a written record of a comprehensive, usually multidisciplinary discussion and reflection on a patient's needs, provides instruction for the VN to take forward. Having been involved with care planning discussions, VNs will have a clear understanding of the goals of care for the patient and allow them to work with autonomy in facilitating those goals. Importantly, having access to a plan of care and associated goals of care may empower nurses to advocate for their patients, should there be a need to adapt care plans and change a course of treatment. Advocacy may be defined as the process by which a nurse speaks out on behalf of their patient. In veterinary nursing this advocacy role may be extended to ensuring the viewpoint of the animal's owner is also put forward.

Care plans may also assist inexperienced veterinary nurses to work independently, within their scope of practice as they follow the planned nursing interventions on the care plan. It may also empower them to approach senior members of the team for help should they reach a point in the care plan they cannot complete without assistance.

Using nursing care plans as a basis to advocate for the best interests of their patients, or to facilitate autonomy and independent practice, will contribute to a greater job satisfaction. VNs will take pride in knowing they have made a difference and have provided care for their patients to the very best of their ability.

A high level of professional satisfaction is a positive emotional response to a job and is one of a range of factors that support high levels of motivation for an occupation. It is motivation that determines how strongly professionals strive to achieve goals. Therefore, it might be assumed that VNs who have increased levels of job satisfaction will work hard to achieve care goals for their patients, potentially achieving improved clinical outcomes.

Nursing care plans and public perception of the role of veterinary nurses

The 2014 RCVS survey of the veterinary nurse profession [1] gathered the opinions of approximately 5400 veterinary nurses, including 1700 student nurses. One of the questions they were asked was what they believed would make their profession better to work within. They were provided with a list of options. The second most-ticked option, after increased pay, was receiving more respect and recognition from the public.

By using nursing care plans and identifying clear nursing interventions that are crucial to the health and wellbeing of animals, veterinary nurses are able to demonstrate their specialised knowledge, unique to their profession. Taking the time to explain a new diagnosis, including the pathophysiology, potential complications, and treatment journey to an owner is a clear demonstration of the knowledge and training the veterinary nurse has and their unique role in facilitating owner understanding. As a therapeutic relationship between nurse and owner develops, the owner will learn more about the role of the nurse within the practice. This has the potential to clarify the role of the VN away from the perception that they are a vet's assistant or a vet in training to the idea that a VN is a professional in their own right with a specific role within the veterinary team.

Nursing care plans and practice revenue

Working to a code of conduct is a characteristic of veterinary nursing that demonstrates it is a recognised profession. The RCVS Code of Conduct in the UK is designed to ensure that the priority of veterinary nurses is always the health and welfare of the animals that have been entrusted to their care. It offers protection for both the animal and the owner of the animal who may be secure in the knowledge that the veterinary nurse is offering care in the best interests of the patient rather than for any financial or professional gain.

With that in mind, it must be acknowledged that veterinary treatment and care is generally supplied to animals as part of a profit-making business. Additionally, a portion of veterinary nurses hold a financial stake in veterinary practices, or at least have some understanding as to the profit and loss status of the business and the importance of financial solvency.

Traditionally, within veterinary practice, veterinary surgeons have always been the sole fee earners. Support staff, including veterinary nurses were considered cost centres, meaning that they were part of the operating costs of a business, but didn't actually contribute to the income at all.

In 2016, the British Veterinary Nursing Association (BVNA) and the RCVS led an initiative to consult with veterinary nurses across the UK on their thoughts and concerns about veterinary nursing, both currently and for the future. The subsequent report, 'VN Futures' [2], identified six clear ambitions for the future of the veterinary nursing profession, each with specific recommendations. One of the ambitions was to 'maximise nurse's potential' and incorporate recognition of skills and the potential that veterinary nurses have to generate income. As part of this ambition there was a recommendation that nurses be encouraged to charge for their professional time and skills.

Veterinary nurses are skilled individuals who can offer services to the owners of animals. A consulting nurse in practice may contribute toward the income of the practice by using a robust and transparent model of charging for the services they offer. Examples include clipping claws, changing wound dressings, applying parasite control, and administering prescribed medication. Veterinary nurses have undergone training and education to be able to carry out these tasks and it is only right that such services should be paid for. Members of the public would not expect to call out a plumber to their leaking tap, only to have it mended for free. Nursing care plans designed to support nursing clinics may assist nurses in setting up clinics and performing consultations. A standardised nursing care plan for clipping claws or assessing a wound may provide structure to the consultation, a tool to facilitate robust record-keeping and potentially a home-care plan so owners may continue the care of the animal at home.

Consider the veterinary care of an animal with a chronic disease, such as diabetes, or renal failure. While facilitating the very best care for that animal, the VN usually provides services that all may be chargeable. Examples include taking and running blood tests, house visits, administering medication, organising repeat prescriptions and weight management. Alongside the direct income that may be created by charging for the services of a nurse, the development of a robust therapeutic relationship where the individual needs of the animal and the owner can be accounted for will increase client loyalty and bonding to a veterinary practice. This may raise the profile of the practice with other members of the local community and likely contribute toward an increased footfall through the business, another potential source of income.

As more and more veterinary nurses run clinics to help owners care for chronically ill patients at home, providing comprehensive home-care plans that also include details of estimated associated costs may help owners plan ahead. They may also help structure a conversation around cost and develop a care plan that is in line with the budget of the owner, potentially resulting in appropriate bills the owner can afford and a reduction in outstanding bad debts and complaints around charging.

Nursing care plans may contribute to effective charging for services provided for an animal while he or she is an inpatient. In the author's experience, it is easy for small items such as food, wound dressings and sterile supplies to be missed when charging for an animal's care. Other chargeable services such as x-rays and blood tests may also be forgotten when they are part of a complex set of care interventions or serial assessments, such as regular ultrasounds. If such omissions are consistent, they may affect practice revenue. A comprehensive nursing care plan should detail the care given so that billing accurately reflects the time and resources used in treating the animal.

Review

- Participating in the care planning process can support veterinary nurses to advocate for their patients.
- The use of nursing care plans can support the professional values of veterinary nursing.
- Clear, contemporary and comprehensive documentation may be a useful tool to support professional accountability.
- Sharing nursing care plans among members of the multidisciplinary team can support collaborative working; however, principles of confidentiality must also be maintained.
- Nursing care plans can have a role in supporting the financial aspect of a veterinary business.

Further reflections

The role of nurses as advocates for their patients is one that is shared between both the human and animal-centred professions. As outlined within this chapter, a nursing care plan, constructed after a participation in the care planning process, can be a valuable tool to support nurses advocating for their patients. When it comes to veterinary nursing, the role of the owner of the animal may be pivotal to the health and welfare of the animal. The owner may often be considered as a member of the extended professional team when decisions about an animals care are being debated. So, given the importance of their role in patient care, should the priority of the veterinary nurse be to act as an advocate for the animal, or for the owner? Think about a situation when you have disagreed with a treatment decision made by an owner. How did it make you feel? Did you advocate for the animal when you believed a poor care decision was being made? Would advocating for that animal have been appropriate in the face of the owner's decision?

References

1. VN Futures Action Group (2016). VN Futures Report.
2. Buzzeo J et al. (2014). The 2014 RCVS Survey of the Veterinary Profession [online]. Last accessed 28th March 2017 at file:///C:/Users/My%20Laptop/Downloads/rcvs-survey-of-the-veterinary-profession-2014%20(1).pdf.

Further reading

These resources offer guidance to professionalism within the human nursing profession, much of which may be applied to veterinary nursing.

1. *Professional Values in Nursing*. Lesley Baillie and Sharon Black (CRC Press, 2015)
2. *The Newly Qualified Nurses Handbook*. Bethann Siviter (Bailliere Tindall, 2008)
3. Nursing and Midwifery *The Code: Professional Standards of Practice and Behaviour for Nurses and Midwives* (NMC, 2015).
4. *Nursing and Working with Other People*. Benny Goodman and Ruth Clemow (Learning Matters, 2008).

Chapter 7

Nursing care plans and clinical governance

By the end of this chapter you will be able to

1. Define and distinguish between clinical governance, clinical effectiveness and clinical audit.
2. Discuss how nursing care plans may be a useful tool to measure care and stimulate research questions.
3. Recognise the potential barriers to using evidence-based practice in veterinary nursing.
4. Provide examples of how using a nursing care plan may assist veterinary nursing education.
5. Discuss how reflective practice may be used to address the gap between the theory of nursing and the practice of nursing.

Clinical governance is an umbrella term for a number of strategies used to recognise and maintain high quality patient care. Fundamentally, it is the process of checking that whatever care is being given is beneficial to the patient and is the best possible care available. It is about keeping patients safe.

There is no single task or policy that demonstrates clinical governance; it may be achieved through the consideration and application of a combination of different factors. Clinical governance should be a culture within a workplace, a culture where questioning and critical thinking is supported. The veterinary team should be encouraged to ask, how good is our practice? How do we know how good our practice is? What can we do to improve our practice?

Clinical governance within veterinary nursing is mandated through the UK RCVS Veterinary Nursing Code of Conduct [1] which clearly states that clinical governance should be part of the veterinary nurse's professional activities.

Clinical governance should incorporate consideration of clinical effectiveness, clinical audit, research and development, education and training, openness, risk management and information management. The effective use of nursing care plans can support several of these factors and subsequently become a valuable tool to support clinical governance.

Features of clinical governance that may be supported by the use of nursing care plans

- Clinical effectiveness
- Clinical audit
- Research and development
- Education and training

Clinical effectiveness

Probably one of the most important factors to support clinical governance is the consideration of the clinical effectiveness of the care provided to patients. **Clinical effectiveness is** defined as a healthcare intervention achieving the expected outcome. It is simply a question of whether the care given worked or not. Clinical effectiveness may support clinical governance in two main ways. First, through the use of evidence-based medicine and second, through the use of clinical audit.

Evidence-based veterinary medicine

When planning the care of a patient, evidence-based interventions should always be considered as first line interventions. **Evidence-based medicine (EBM)** is described as an integration of the use of the best research available with clinical expertise and patient values and circumstances. These are principles laid down by David Sackett within the context of human medicine in the 1990s.

Clinical expertise is assumed to be the proficiency and judgement that individual clinicians acquire through clinical experience and practice. The best research available should be clinically relevant, and, if possible, incorporate data obtained through meta-analysis of well-designed randomised controlled trials or be strong evidence from a systematic review. Within human-centred medicine, an example of an ideal research source would be information obtained from a Cochrane review.

One of the strongest criticisms of evidence-based practice is that it is pre-prescribed medicine, colloquially referred to as cookbook medicine, that dictates how patients should be treated. In contrast, the three elements of evidence-based medicine best research, clinical expertise and patient values and circumstances, defy that opinion and encourage the use of EBM in an objective way, guiding healthcare professionals to consider the external factors that make patients and, in the case of veterinary medicine, owners unique. Nursing models of care provide guidance as to the factors that make up the individual circumstances and values of a patient. The Orpet and Jeffery Ability Model [2] advocates consideration of the owners culture and ability to adhere to patient care instructions, as well as ensuring that the financial situation of the owner is also taken into account. Care must be applied and evaluated constantly. The very best evidence-based practice is no good repeated over and over again if it is not effective. VNs must be confident to think laterally and use the veterinary nursing process and their clinical expertise to structure their care and evaluate, adjust and adapt their care plans as necessary.

The use of evidence-based practice has several advantages, most importantly, the use of proven clinical interventions supports the aim of providing clinically effective care. It may improve care and reduce time wasted on inappropriate and ineffective clinical interventions.

The use of evidence-based practice may also benefit the owner of the animal. It promotes cost effectiveness as resources may be directed carefully and appropriately for interventions that have been proven to be clinically effective.

The use of evidence-based practice supports the veterinary nurse in their practice. Veterinary nurses are personally accountable for their professional actions and practicing evidence-based medicine may facilitate the VNs' ability to explain and justify their clinical decisions.

Benefits of using evidence-based practice in veterinary nursing

1. Improved clinical outcomes
2. Effective use of resources
3. Promotion of professional accountability

Within veterinary nursing there are three significant barriers to the consistent application of evidence-based practice. Primarily, there is simply a lack of evidence to support veterinary nursing care interventions within the profession. There is a wealth of human-centred nursing evidence that may be borrowed or adapted, but little specific to veterinary nursing. Fortunately, this situation is improving, through a combination of the publishing of veterinary nursing specific peer reviewed journals and an increase in graduate veterinary nurses who are more familiar with critiquing, appraising and carrying out primary research and sharing their skills with the practice team.

The increased use of veterinary nursing specific care plans is a demonstration of evidence-based veterinary nursing. More and more nurses are using a structured approach to nursing care as evidence continues to build that doing so promotes holistic individualised and effective care.

Cost may also be a significant barrier to the use of evidence-based practice, both professionally and clinically. Professionally, it has been proven that veterinary nurses often support their own continuing professional development both with their own money and their own time. At a recent educational event, chaired by the author, a survey of attendees revealed that approximately 75% of them had paid for themselves to attend the course. In 2015, the British Veterinary Nursing Association [3] surveyed a thousand of their members and learned that 92% of them paid for their own membership. This demonstrates an actively engaged profession, but also a profession who are not necessarily familiar with having continual professional development activities paid for them. It may be assumed that the same principles apply to membership subscriptions for journals, research databases or veterinary libraries. Therefore, veterinary nurses may well be reliant on providing their own evidence-based resources, a daunting prospect for a professional only just beginning to grapple with applying evidence in practice.

Clinically, the costs of care may prohibit the care that can be administered which may prevent the best evidence-based practice being implemented to save costs for an owner. This can be difficult for the professional team to accept. It demonstrates how important the care planning process is, as the financial factor may be taken into account and options presented to the owner of the best evidence-based practice, within their stated budget, so that the owner is not under any obligation to extend their financial circumstances beyond their means.

Finally, and most simply, the owner of the animal may choose not to consent to the best evidence-based intervention and opt for a different approach. This may be due to cultural or compliance factors. So, while the evidence may suggest that a polypharmacy medical approach to a health problem is more effective than the surgical option, both should be presented and the owner supported in their decision, even if they opt for the inferior surgical option. The reasons for their decision should be explored; for example, the prospect of giving the animal tablets might be too much for an owner and therefore, out of the two options, the surgery is the most appealing.

Barriers to the use of evidence-based practice in veterinary nursing

1. Availability and accessibility of evidence
2. Professional and patient costs
3. Owner choice

Measuring care

While the use of evidence-based practice may support the aim of providing clinically effective treatment it is the measurement of care that determines clinical effectiveness. The measurement of care may be controversial. Historically, the process of caring has been a vocational and noble act. Anecdotally, the characteristics of a good nurse may be linked to key personality traits such as a caring nature, being kind and compassionate, and in possession of an excellent ability to communicate clearly and concisely. It is these personality-linked traits that may make the measurement of nursing care controversial, as it may be interpreted as the measurement and judgement of a personality rather than a professional role. However, the measurement of clinical outcomes of nursing interventions is essential to support clinical governance and check that patients are receiving care that is appropriate for them and their situation.

Clinical audit

The use of a clinical audit is a key tool in the measurement of care. A clinical audit may be defined as a measurement of clinical care compared to an agreed standard. Essentially, a clinical audit is a method of measuring a very specific element of healthcare with the aim of finding out whether the care is performed in the very best way. Carrying out an audit is a cyclical process, a process that may be demonstrated through a series of questions that must be answered (Figure 7.1).

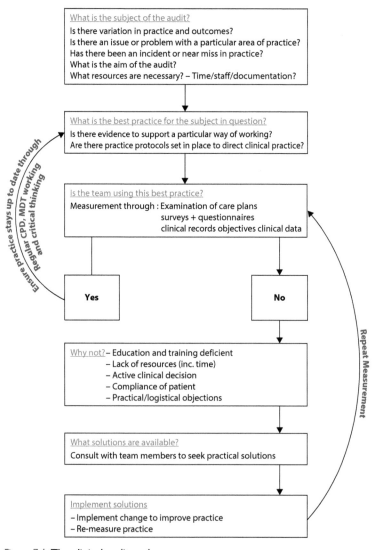

Figure 7.1 **The clinical audit cycle.**

The comprehensive record-keeping that is stimulated through the use of nursing care plans may support clinical audit activities in practice. Through the use of a nursing model, attention to details, for example, the diet an animal receives while hospitalised, are all recorded within a comprehensive and holistic care plan, regardless of the reason the animal requires treatment.

The use of a specific diet is a good example of implementing an audit within the practice (Figure 7.2). As an example, a retrospective study based on the information from nursing care plans may reveal that the nurses within a practice all tend to use a particular type of food when feeding animals after a general anaesthetic. There are specific diets that are useful for post-operative feeding, however, the clinical audit, demonstrates that the diet that has the most evidence attached to it is not actually being selected by the team. This process allows the team to allows the team to ask why the diet is not being used and potentially implement strategies to support the use of best practice.

Within human-centred medicine, the National Institute for Health Care and Excellence (NICE) produces national clinical guidelines, technological appraisals, social and staffing guidance for human-centred medicine on a huge range of conditions, symptoms, patient groups and healthcare environments. Based on the expertise of medical professionals, technical experts and representatives from patient groups, these may form the backbone of most clinical audits and are a vast source of evidence-based guidance.

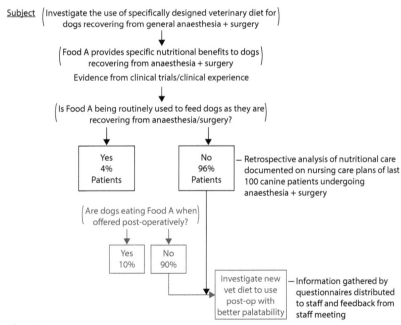

Figure 7.2 In practice – Clinical audit example.

In practice – The use of NICE guidelines in clinical audit

The NICE guidelines for the prevention of pressure ulcers in adults (CG179) within human-centred nursing are clear that all patients should be risk assessed for pressure ulcers on admission to hospital [4]. Furthermore, they should be reassessed should their clinical condition change. The guidance also suggests that a standardised assessment tool is used in this risk assessment. These simple guidelines may be used within an audit of pressure ulcer care on a hospital ward. The baseline may be established that every patient on the ward should have been risk assessed for pressure ulcers. An audit of clinical records can be carried out to establish whether that is happening. Each chart can be checked to see whether it contains reference to pressure ulcer risk assessment, or alternatively, a documented reason as to why it might not have been completed with the recommended assessment tool. It may be established that 100% of the patients had been assessed for their risk of developing pressure ulcers, but only 80% of the patients that day had been assessed using the recommended assessment tool. The reason cited for 10% of patients being assessed without using the assessment tool was that the pressure ulcer assessment forms had run out and there were none available on the ward. The nurses had deemed their patients to be independently mobile and therefore able to relieve their own pressure areas. So, completing this tool had been moved down the priority list of care needs.

In this somewhat simplistic example, there is a quick fix, to ensure that there are always enough assessment tools on the ward. It might be worth exploring if the necessary documentation was moved online whether it would improve staff access to them. Or perhaps a member of the administration team might be put in charge of ensuring the relevant paperwork was always available. Whatever the possible solution, the audit stimulates identification of issues so that possible solutions may be suggested.

As has been discussed, establishing an evidence-based standard for the baseline of a clinical audit within veterinary nursing may be significantly more difficult than in human-centred nursing, but not impossible. Instead of relying exclusively on evidence from meta-analysis or randomised controlled trials, the clinical team within a practice may develop their own standardised clinical protocols. After all, there are some areas of veterinary nursing where it would be unethical to test clinical effectiveness. Establishing standardised clinical protocols within a veterinary practice may be a suitable starting point to measure effective practice.

Research

Research and development is another element of clinical governance. Clinical research is the name given to the process of developing new healthcare related practice. In comparison to a clinical audit, research strives to produce new knowledge and test it to see if it works. Research may be stimulated when it is noticed that there is a gap in the knowledge, and there is no literature or clinical knowledge to fill that gap. Potentially, the results of a clinical audit may become the basis of new research projects as nurses try and establish methods of working to overcome any deficits in care identified by an audit.

Never has there been a better time in the history of veterinary nursing for members of the profession to try and develop research projects. A combination of the need for professional accountability, an increasing number of VNs with the necessary skills coming into the profession, and a desire to push the profession forward all combine to create an environment ripe for the development of new ideas in veterinary nursing care.

The use of nursing care plans supports holistic care. It is this model of working that may improve the knowledge associated with a condition or a set of symptoms. There is a greater awareness of the whole animal and therefore a greater awareness of the other factors that may affect animal health as well as physical changes. Through the identification of trends from information obtained via a thorough and detailed assessment shared traits may be identified. A simple example would be cats suffering from Feline Lower Urinary Tract Disease (FLUTD). Over time, the profession has been able to identify that cats with certain characteristics are overrepresented with this condition, for example, those who are subjected to stress, kept indoors, are overweight and/or neutered.

Education and training

The use of nursing care plans may also support education and training, which is another principle of clinical governance. Veterinary nurses cannot be expected to provide high quality care without undergoing specific education and training. Nursing care plans feature in current veterinary nursing training. Student nurses are taught the fundamentals of human-centred nursing theory and how it may be applied to veterinary patients. VNs need to understand how to use a care plan to optimise the care of their patients, taking account actual and potential nursing needs. They need to be encouraged to contribute to the care planning process with colleagues and learn how to review a care plan systematically.

Examples of robust nursing care plans may be used to inform student nurses on the principles of care planning and how a care plan may benefit clinical practice. Experienced nurses may be guilty of assuming that nursing care plans are only ever useful as educational tools to direct inexperienced nurses in the care of their patients. This is narrow-minded, as while nursing care plans may be useful teaching tools and may empower inexperienced nurses to be advocates for their patients, they have multiple benefits for experienced nurses as well. The professional benefits of nursing care plans apply across the entire demographic of the nursing team. The support of professional accountability, improved perception of the veterinary nurse, and development of research ideas all apply to experienced nurses. Care plans are a useful aide memoir for a busy team, ensuring patient needs are not missed. Experience cannot be relied upon all day every day. Human beings are fallible and therefore, a care plan may help avoid mistakes and compromise of patient safety should care needs be inadvertently missed.

Reflective practice

One of the best examples of using nursing care plans for nursing education is to combine them with education on reflective practice. Reflective practice is a key aspect of human-centred nursing care. In fact, in the UK, demonstration of evidence that nurses are working as reflective practitioners is a mandatory requirement when human-centred nurses renew their registration with the Nursing and Midwifery Council, a process known as revalidation [5]. They are required to demonstrate to another NMC registered nurse, known as a confirmer, that they have five written reflections that have influenced their clinical practice. They must participate in a reflective discussion with their confirmer and be able to link both their discussion and their written reflections to aspects of the NMC code of conduct.

Reflective practice is a process whereby critical incidents are considered in a structured and thoughtful way. **A critical incident may** be defined as any event that stimulates a reaction for the nurse, be it good or bad. There are many ways of structuring reflection, mainly through cyclical tools that guide the process. However, the key theme is that nurses are encouraged to extract learning outcomes from their thought process and develop their practice.

When it comes to nursing education, reflective practice is also an essential method of addressing the potential gap between the theory of nursing and the reality, the practical, clinical nursing. Nursing students, both human and veterinary centred, can be taught how to write excellent, comprehensive care plans that use prime evidence-based practice while in the classroom. However, it is possible that once in practice, they may struggle to implement such prescriptive care plans and this can lead to confusion and anxiety.

Reflection on a critical incident may allow the teacher or lecturer to explain external factors that may influence a nursing care plan. Factors such as those that have been described in this text, and highlighted by Orem, RLT, and Orpet and Jeffery, including owner compliance and financial and cultural considerations, may all mean that veterinary staff are unable to implement the ideal evidence-based practice. Being able to reason this through and understand why evidence-based practice cannot always be applied can help students to understand how to apply evidence-based practice. It may support them to understand how they must strive to implement evidence-based practice, but always take into account the animal and the owner to ensure that it suits them and their situation.

Review

- Clinical governance is an umbrella term for a number of strategies that can be put in place to ensure that standards of clinical practice are optimal.
- Using evidence-based practice may promote optimal standards of clinical practice, but it must be used within the context of the individual patient and applied with the consideration of clinical experience and judgement.
- Clinical audits are a useful tool to support clinical governance and may also act as a springboard for further research and development.
- Reflective practice is a crucial element of human-centred nursing and is likely to become just as important in veterinary nursing. It promotes learning and development and can also be a tool to address the potential gap between learned theory and practical nursing.

Further reflections

In the UK, the Royal College of Veterinary Surgeons regulate veterinary nursing through the Veterinary Nursing Code of Conduct. This code of conduct is explicit about clinical governance mandating that all veterinary nurses should participate in activities to support clinical governance.

Read the code of conduct. Are there any further parts of the code that also relate to the principles of clinical governance more implicitly?

Consider the practice in which you work. Can you identify tasks or actions that link into the principles of clinical governance? If so, list them and consider how many you are directly involved in. If not, consider whether there are any recent issues or topics that are being discussed that might benefit from application of an audit to generate robust practice-specific data. Enlist the support of one of your veterinary colleagues and plan an audit using the audit cycle.

References

1. Royal College of Veterinary Surgeons (2014). Code of Professional Conduct for Veterinary Nurses [online]. Last accessed 28th March 2017. http://www.rcvs.org .uk/advice-and-guidance/code-of-professional-conduct-for-veterinary-nurses/.
2. Orpet H and Welsh P (2011). *Handbook of Veterinary Nursing*. 2nd ed. Oxford: Wiley-Blackwell.
3. British Veterinary Nursing Association (2015). Survey of Members.
4. National Institute of Health and Care Excellence (2014). Pressure Ulcers: Preventions and Management [online]. Last accessed 28th March 2017. https://www.nice.org.uk/Guidance/ CG179.
5. Nursing and Midwifery Council (2016). Welcome to Revalidation [online]. Last accessed 19th September 2016. http://revalidation.nmc.org.uk/welcome-to-revalidation.

Further reading

Practical resources are available to assist in establishing easy and accessible clinical governance and reflective practice.

1. Clinical Audit Tool Kit www.knowledge.rcvs.org.uk.
2. NHS England – A guide to clinical audit https://www.england.nhs.uk/ourwork/qual-clin-lead/ clinaudit/.
3. *Reflective Practice in Nursing*. Linda Howatson-Jones (Learning Matters, 2011).
4. *Nursing Standard* – Weekly nursing journal which publishes reflections from student and qualified nurses in every edition.
5. *The Evidence-Based Practice Manual for Nurses*, 3rd edition. Jean V Craig and Rosalind L Smyth (Churchill Livingstone Elsevier, 2012).
6. *Doing Your Research Project:* A Guide for First Time Researchers in Education Health and Social Science, 5th edition. Judith Bell (Open University Press, 2010).

Section III

How to use nursing care plans in practice

Chapter 8

Writing nursing care plans

By the end of this chapter you will be able to

1. Identify the different types of nursing care plans used in human-centred nursing.
2. Evaluate the advantages and disadvantages of different types of care plans.
3. List the characteristics of a well written care plan.
4. Use SMART principles to compose goals of care.
5. Define and apply the principles of critical thinking.
6. Design a nursing care plan using the veterinary nursing process in combination with models of nursing care.

Combining the use of nursing models with the nursing process provides structure to nursing care. It stimulates a comprehensive, holistic assessment which, when analysed in the context of the individual situation of the patient, stimulates a plan of care which can be documented.

Guidelines for writing nursing care plans

There are clear guidelines as to how nursing documentation, which includes nursing care plans, should be managed from both the UK's Nursing and Midwifery Council and the Royal College of Veterinary Surgeons (RCVS). The overall emphasis from the RCVS is clear: the code of conduct for veterinary nurses in the UK states that 'veterinary nurses must keep clear, accurate and detailed clinical nursing and client records' [1].

Further advice guides veterinary professionals to document any information they provide to an owner, also advising that entries they make should be objective. Any records should avoid personal observations or assumptions about a client's motivation, financial circumstances or other matters. So, while it might be appropriate to document an agreed financial limit on the care plan, it is not likely to be appropriate to document personal opinions on why owners have agreed to such a limit.

There is also guidance for amending nursing documentation. If a care plan is in need of an adjustment due to error, the original entry should not be obliterated, but should have a line drawn through it. Additionally, the details of the person making the adjustment must be clear to see.

Nursing care plans may be presented in many different formats, but there are universal characteristics all care plans should share. Ideally, care plans should be written in permanent black ink to promote longevity and facilitate electronic reproduction if necessary. All care plans should be clearly marked with the details of the patient it refers to. It is important to ensure that all pages of a care plan are clearly labelled with the patient details, even if the care plan is double-sided.

Consider that if the document should be photocopied onto individual, single-sided sheets, as it would be easy for the second unlabelled sheet to be lost.

Within human centred healthcare, it is mandated that staff members check four points of identification: first name, surname, date of birth and identification number, before a nursing intervention is carried out. Clearly with animals this is difficult, as an animal cannot provide a full name and date of birth. The animal's name and owners surname should be clearly displayed on the care plan. Consideration should also be given to the use of other points of identification, like naming the breed and providing a description of the animal's appearance. In some practices paper collars with a patient's name and identification number are used to ensure clear points of identity are available.

As well as clear identification of the patient the care plan refers to, there is need for clear identification of the nurse writing the care plan. Every entry should be signed with a signature, corresponding printed name, and the date and time the entry was made.

Care plans should display details of the intended nursing interventions for the patient. It is also useful to provide details of the assessment and goals of the care so that the team are united in the aims of caring for the patient. If novel or unfamiliar procedures are being carried out on the patient, there should be consideration of the addition of diagrams, flow charts or instructions to facilitate staff understanding.

Guidelines for writing care plans

1. Use permanent black ink.
2. Label the care plan with the relevant patient details (both sides of the sheet).
3. Sign, date and time all entries.
4. List the interventions the patient needs and the goals of the planned care.
5. Be creative and use additional diagrams or instructions if indicated.
6. Avoid the use of abbreviations unless they have been agreed upon within the nursing team.
7. Use clear and concise language.
8. Read the care plan before finishing to ensure it is clear and error free.

Developing goals of care

Most nursing models advocate using goals of care, however, they offer little guidance as to how they might be structured and designed. Setting goals of care falls under the planning stage of the nursing process. The primary care goal may be to return an animal back to health. However, this is likely to require many smaller interventions, for example, administration of medication, the use of wound dressings, a surgical procedure or a specific diet.

Goals may be separated into long and short term goals of care. Short-term goals generally concentrate on addressing the patient's clinical symptoms, working to a broader, longer term goal, such as returning an animal to work or getting them home to the family. Goal planning should also address both actual and potential problems. The role of the nurse is not limited to simply treating problems. There is a need to ensure health promotion and facilitate the treatment of animals to ensure that the same problem does not reoccur.

In practice – Setting goals

Jonas is a one-year-old domestic short hair cat who has presented to the practice unable to urinate. The goals of his care may be broken down into three sections: priority care, supportive therapy and maintenance of health.

The priority care goals would be to treat any pain or discomfort, facilitate the free flow of urine and normalise any electrolyte imbalance that he has suffered as a result of his condition. Once these goals have been met, the next stage of treatment may continue. Goals for supportive therapy are likely to involve supporting urinary flow through use of medications and establishing a cause for his symptoms.

Finally, once the acute phase of the illness has been resolved, the final set of care goals is linked to the maintenance of health. Goals would include ensuring the owner knows the signs and symptoms that might signal recurrence. They also need to understand and be able to implement measures that can be taken to prevent recurrence.

Specific, measurable, achievable, realistic and timed goals

The SMART (specific, measurable, achievable, realistic and timed) model is a useful standardised format for planning goals. Used widely, and applicable to most situations, including project planning, it is a simple and effective way of writing goals that are useful and appropriate.

Specific

Goals of care need to be specific; they should describe the desired outcome in a focused and well-defined way. If possible, to promote an objective view, the outcome should be related to a number, a percentage, fraction or frequency.

Measurable

The planned goal of care should have some form of measurable outcome so that a judgment can be made on whether it has been achieved or not. Again, to support a truly objective goal, where possible, the measurement should have a numerical element. If the goal is truly qualitative, then specific markers of achievement should be set.

Achievable

To assess whether a goal of care is achievable, questions must be asked. Can the goal actually be met? Has it been done before? Are there any direct contraindications to doing it?

Realistic

At this stage, patient-specific factors should be taken into account to assess whether the goal is actually appropriate for the patient in question. Usually goals of care are demanding, and require input from the patient and, in veterinary nursing, the owner, but they should not be overly demanding and therefore unachievable. The RLT model in human-centred nursing highlights the emphasis of a patient's culture, politics, economic and psychological status as potentially having a direct impact on nursing care. In veterinary nursing, the Ability Model advocates the consideration of the culture and financial status of the owner while the animal is an inpatient and the likely compliance of the owner in facilitating further care to the animal within the home environment. So, another series of questions must be asked of the planned goal. Does the veterinary team have the relevant skills and expertise? Does the owner agree that this is an appropriate goal for the animal? Does the owner have the necessary resources to support the interventions to achieve this goal?

Timing

Finally, goals should include a date or time by which they will be accomplished or completed. Within healthcare the timing of the goal may be selected to coincide with the end of a course of medication or therapy. Additionally, within healthcare the use of review dates is important. Review dates are an additional marker of the progress of a goal of care. They are usually interim dates, set before the goal is expected to be achieved when care maybe evaluated to ensure that improvements are being made. If not, reassessment might be indicated. Review dates are used on drug charts throughout the NHS so all members of the multidisciplinary team are encouraged to support the appropriate use of antibiotics. A review date triggers a microbiology review to ensure that the drugs being given are relevant to the problem identified.

Consider the example of the nutritional care goal (Figure 8.1), while this is a relatively lengthy example, it could be shortened when used within the context of a busy working

Using SMART principles to plan a nutritional care goal

– GEORGE is a 7-year-old labrador suffering from diarrhoea and vomiting.

– Nutritional goal

Ensure George has food
Offer food little and often   X

Unanswered questions

What food should George have?
How often should he have food?
How much food should he have?
What if he is sick after eating his food?

Nutritional goal – according to SMART principles

Specific	– Aim to provide George with X kilocalories over 24 hours (stating 0900 23/3/17) – Feed XX grams of food every 2 hours – Monitor response to food
Measurable	– Document kcals consumed to enable review of intake
Achievable	– 24-hour nursing available – Chicken available (George's favourite)
Realistic	– George has already eaten 50 g of chicken so likely to eat more – Owner happy with plan and bringing in alternative favourite foods in case George doesn't eat chicken.
Timed	– Reassess kcal intake total every 6 hours and report to vet if George not expected to achieve full intake of kcal.

Figure 8.1 In practice – Nutritional care goal set according to SMART principles.

day. It is a goal that should last for 24 hours and makes provision for re-evaluation and adaptation should the patient's clinical status change, for example if he starts refusing oral intake. Compare this goal of care to the frequently recorded nutritional plan of 'feeding little and often'. A goal and plan of care constructed with SMART principles in mind provides much more detail and includes objective measurements of progress through measurement of kilocalories taken in over a set number of hours. It is this detail that will support continuity of care and ensure that the nursing team understand and work towards the same goal of care. When writing out SMART goals is prohibited by timing constraints, the SMART principles remain a useful framework to think through care goals and ensure they are as useful as possible.

Freehand nursing care plans

Human-centred nursing has a longer history of using care plans than veterinary nursing. There are subsequently two basic formats of care plan that have been developed, each with their own advantages and disadvantages. Generalised nursing care plans are written freehand for each patient where details of the planned care may be written under the headings, problem, goals and interventions, or simply under the nursing process headings, assessment, plan, nursing diagnosis intervention and evaluation. These enable detailed records to be kept for each individual and will encourage the inclusion of details specific to that patient and their family. They can also be an excellent tool for communicating novel treatment plans that colleagues may not be familiar with as the freehand aspect will encourage the use of diagrams, mind mapping, step by step instructions and references to evidence.

In contrast, it might be argued that without use of a clear model or structure for the assessment, the nursing team might lack direction and patient care might be compromised. It would be easy to concentrate on the problem the patient is presenting with, inadvertently reverting to the medical model rather than conducting a full holistic assessment. Furthermore, such care plans are often time-consuming as nurses struggle within a busy shift to structure their care plan logically and methodically.

A useful structure to format such freehand care plans is the use of SOAP, which stands for, subjective observations, objective observations, assessment, and plan. The example (Figure 8.2) illustrates a patient's care plan written by nurse (TA) for another nurse to facilitate during the day shift. In the example, after completing the care, the second nurse (KK) completes documentation of her actions. She confirms that she has worked with the patient to facilitate their understanding of their new medication. **Subjectively,** she reports that the patient asked appropriate questions, demonstrating his engagement with the process. **Objectively,** she reports that the patient was able to select the correct drug and dose, demonstrating his ability to manage his own warfarin administration. Her **assessment** overall is that he is confident in managing his warfarin independently. Finally, his future care **plan** is documented, the plan to provide further support at home from his local care team via his general practitioner.

Standardised care plans

An alternative to freehand generalised nursing care plan are the standardised care plans used within human-centred nursing. Usually they are designed for specific problems or care needs and therefore, each patient may need several care plans throughout their care episode. These care plans

Please affix patient label or complete details below

Full name: DAVE

Hospital number:

NHS number:

DOB: 27/04/1960

Papworth Hospital NHS

NHS Foundation Trust

Care Plan

Ward 3

Problem/need

BEGIN WARFARIN / ANTI-COAGULANT THERAPY POST PULMONARY EMBOLISM

Aim/goal

Self care – patient to understand treatment and associated monitoring, risks and drug/food interactions

Plan PLAN FOR DAY SHIFT NURSE 25/3/17

✓ 1. Resources – leaflet / monitoring chart / warfarin card

✓ 2. Refer to local anticoagulant clinic

✓ 3. Explain treatment – side effects / potential complications; explain INR / blood tests; interactions warfarin + food + drugs

✓ 4. Arrange / refer to pharmacist for warfarin counselling.

S Warfarin treatment covered in discussion with patient + family (wife). He asked appropriate questions, demonstrated comprehension of side

O effects and accurate selection of correct drug and correct dose

P Referral completed for warfarin clinic at patient's GP

A Dave happy with plan to attend GP 28/3/17., Confident in managing his own warfarin

(KK) Kim Kitty Staff Nurse 25/3/17

Date 24/3/17 Time 23:00 Initial TA Signature

Print name Tim Alfreddo Designation Staff Nurse

ND 35 Blank Care Plan. V2. File section 4. Review 08/2014

Figure 8.2 Human-centred freehand nursing care plan. (Reproduced from Papworth Hospital NHS Foundation Trust. With kind permission.)

utilise the fact that although patients are all unique in their care needs, there will be similarities in the treatments that are offered and implemented. So, two patients with surgical wounds may have had completely different surgery and will have different rates of healing, and different factors affecting their healing. However, the wounds both need dressing to support healing, so nurses must know what dressing has been used previously, what the wound looked like the last time it was examined and what medication might support the wound. In having access to all this information, the nurse can evaluate the care given with the aim of establishing if progress is being made. If the wound looks worse than it did when the last nurse described it, there is need for a change in the care plan, a new dressing or new medication. While the list of factors to consider may be standardised, the ability to tick boxes, or add freehand comments makes it individual to that patient.

There are several benefits to such a tool. First, guidance may be provided within the document including key evidence-based interventions that patients may need. Examples of such standardised care plans include the use of oxygen therapy and the treatment of pyrexia. Both stimulate the nurse to carry out specific tasks to offer the best possible care. In using a standardised care plan to treat low oxygen saturations, (Figure 8.3) nurses are reminded to titrate the oxygen according to the oxygen saturation measurements and continue to monitor the patient.

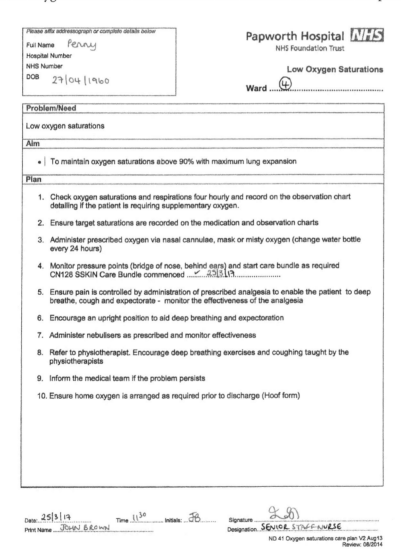

Figure 8.3 Human-centred standardised nursing care plan. (Reproduced from Papworth Hospital NHS Foundation Trust. With kind permission.)

(Continued)

	Please affix addressograph or complete details below		Papworth Hospital **NHS**

Please affix addressograph or complete details below

Full Name *Penny*

Hospital Number

NHS Number

DOB *27|04|60*

Papworth Hospital **NHS**
NHS Foundation Trust

Low Oxygen Saturations

Ward ......④...

Date	Time	Care Plan/Evaluation	Signature / Print/ Designation
25/3/17	11³⁰	Care plan started after observations revealed low O2 – 89%. No other symptoms of concern, other observation within range for patient. Assisted patient to chair with immediate improvement. Referral to physiotherapy for deep breathing exercise, review analgesia, pain score 0 currently.	JOHN BROWN SENIOR STAFF NURSE.
25/3/17	14⁴⁰	O2 saturations at 93% no O2 supplementary required.	

Date:.............................   Time .... Initials: ....   Signature ....

Print Name ....   Designation..

ND 41 Oxygen saturations care plan V2 Aug13
Review: 08/2014

Figure 8.3 (Continued) **Human-centred standardised nursing care plan. (Reproduced from Papworth Hospital NHS Foundation Trust. With kind permission.)**

Second, these types of care plans may be excellent tools for supporting inexperienced nurses, as reading and using the care plan may direct their actions.

Third, they are very often proposed to be time-saving devices, one example being supporting a patient's personal hygiene needs. Many hospitalised patients require assistance to wash themselves. A care plan that is pre-printed with the basic elements of assisting with personal care may save a nurse writing out their precise actions, step by step. There must always be space for extra comment and adaptation, to ensure the individualism is not lost but the nurse is spared the timely need to repeat the same narrative for each and every patient they care for (Figure 8.4).

Please affix patient label or complete details below		
Full name: *Judy*		
Hospital number:		
NHS number:		
DOB: *27/04/1960*		

Papworth Hospital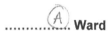
NHS Foundation Trust

Washing and Dressing

............(A).. **Ward**

Problem/need
...*Judy*........ is currently unable to maintain own standard of hygiene.
Aim/goal
Standards of hygiene are maintained until the patient is independent
Plan
1. Assess ability to maintain own hygiene
2. Offer full assisted wash, assisted shower, assisted bath as required
3. Ensure use of disposable wash cloths and 2 towels
4. Do bath temperatures as per hospital protocol
5. Offer hand washing after toileting and prior to meals
6. Offer patient additional wash in the evening
7. Encourage patient when independent to use shower instead of bath
8. Ensure post transplant patients do not use hospital showers
9. Ensure wash bowls / baths are thoroughly cleaned after each patient
10. Ensure hair, nail and mouth-care is given
11. Offer mouthcare to patients pre bed unable to access bathrooms
12. Maintain dignity and privacy at all times

Date *23/3/17* Time *14⁰⁰* Initial *JB* Signature *JB)*

Print name *JOHN BROWN* Designation *SENIOR STAFF NURSE*

ND 92 Washing and dressing V2. File section 4. Review: 12/2014

Figure 8.4 Completed human-centred standardised nursing care plan. (Reproduced from Papworth Hospital NHS Foundation Trust. With kind permission.)

(Continued)

Date	Time	Care Plan / Evaluation	Signature/Print/ designation
24/3/17	10⁰⁰	Care provided according to care plan – patient has own toiletries with him – prefers showers – never has baths at home.	J.B. JOHN BROWN SENIOR STAFF NURSE

Figure 8.4 (Continued) Completed human-centred standardised nursing care plan. (Reproduced from Papworth Hospital NHS Foundation Trust. With kind permission.)

However, such nursing care plans are usually very specific to certain symptoms or sets of symptoms which may inadvertently mean that other care needs are given less attention, or even missed. It is possible that pre-printed care plans may send nursing back into the very medical model of nursing that the theorists of the 1960s and 1970s strove to move away from. Such specific nursing care plans must be used in the context of a full assessment to ensure individualised, relevant care. A wound, no matter how well dressed, will not heal in an immunosuppressed patient, with deranged glucose levels and poor nutrition. In reality, such nursing care plans are indeed put into place after a full assessment and while this helps to ensure a holistic approach, it makes for a paperwork-heavy admission if each nursing intervention requires its own individual care plan.

Critical thinking

It is only right that veterinary nurses look to their human-centred counterparts for ideas and inspiration on ways of working. There are lessons to be learned from both the triumphs and mistakes of the human-centred nursing profession. There is a wealth of information, opinion and evidence that is available for consideration on many different aspects of nursing. But, veterinary nursing as a profession cannot and should not blindly adopt theory and policy simply because it works for human-centred nurses. Veterinary nurses must think about it, analyse it, practice it, talk about it and examine it. In essence, they must apply critical thinking to it. **Critical thinking** is the application of a questioning attitude to practice. It involves using a combination of experience, intellect, and emotion to draw conclusions that may be acted on in a professional manner. It is easy to follow instructions and perform tasks without ever asking why. Thinking critically may promote patient health and patient safety.

As an example, many animals do not like going to the veterinary practice, but animals with chronic health problems need to have regular examinations from the veterinary team so that supportive care may be managed and legal obligations are fulfilled for continued prescribing of medication. Critical thinking can help to develop new practice and services for animals and their owners. A nurse who is thinking critically would never think, 'They have to bring this animal in every two weeks, because that's the way we always do things here'. In contrast, they would think carefully, and potentially try and adapt their practice to make meeting the care needs of the animal easier for the owner. They may consider offering an appointment at the weekend, a telephone consultation or less frequent examinations. However, if it is indeed essential that the animal is seen every two weeks, that same nurse, thinking critically, will discuss it openly with the owner and talk through their difficulties and offer explanation and support. If an owner is able to understand why care is needed and what care goals the team are trying to achieve, they are more likely to work to facilitate them.

In practice – Critical thinking

Consider the following instruction to administer medication to an animal. The instruction reads 'Give 50 mg medication X twice daily with food.' What happens if the nurse goes to collect that medication from the pharmacy and they find out that medication X only comes in 1 mg tablets? A nurse thinking critically would question this, as essentially following those instructions would involve administrating fifty individual tablets to the animal. Surely that is unusual enough to speak to the prescribing vet and double check the dose and the medication?

The in-practice example demonstrates that critical thinking is not about challenging colleagues, but simply about thinking things through and not making assumptions.

Writing nursing care plans

The actual designing and writing of a nursing care plan will vary from practice to practice, potentially from animal to animal. However, there is a similar process that may be used to create the document. It is a process that combines the guidelines for nursing documentation, as provided by the relevant regulatory bodies, with the use of nursing models and the nursing process. Throughout the development of the care plan, critical thinking is essential to ensure the document is useful to both the nurse and the patient.

Figure 8.5 provides clear guidance as to where the elements discussed throughout this textbook fit into actually writing a relevant and useful care plan. Nursing models are used within the veterinary nursing process to provide direction and detail to the assessment and therefore the evaluation of the care. The care plan is the documentation of planned interventions. When used in a contemporary manner and adjusted and adapted as patient needs change, it can support both patient care and the nursing team who are working to a specific professional code of conduct.

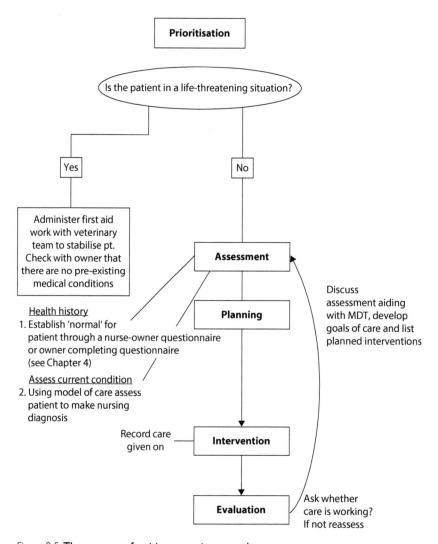

Figure 8.5 The process of writing a nursing care plan.

Within the context of veterinary nursing, there are two ways to apply nursing care plans practically. First, they may be used as a tool to guide assessment. They may be stand-alone documents that nurses can use intermittently to guide their clinical decision-making, ensuring that all patient needs are met and a record of the care planning process is recorded (Figure 8.6).

Such documents are clear and easy to read, facilitating access to patient information to all members of the multidisciplinary team. They are also a useful tool when a practice is starting to introduce formal care planning as they provide clear direction as to how the care planning assessment may be carried out.

Alternatively, the nursing care plan can be combined with the record of patient observations, commonly known as the hospitalisation sheet. This has the advantage of reducing the amount of paperwork associated with patient care and provides a real-time update and evaluation of care as objective and subjective data is recorded and the care plan is adjusted implicitly (Figure 8.7).

PATIENT NAME _Sandy_
OWNER NAME _Smith_
BREED _Labrador X_
AGE _11 Years_

DIAGNOSIS
Pyometra
(Confirmed via ultrasound)

Activity of living	Home/Normal	Current	Intervention	Signature
1. Maintaining safe environment	Family pet lives in house with family	1—	None	25/3/17 1430 Fiona Andrew
2. Communicating (owner)	Owner by family	Kennels brought in Sandy – owners on holiday.	Will need written care instructions for owner	25/3/17 1430 Fiona Andrew
3. Breathing	No concerns	None	None	25/3/17 Fiona Andrew
4. Eating and drinking	Body score 5 dry food, twice daily	Not eaten since 4 PM 24/3/17	Starve pre-surgery do nutritional plan for recovery	25/3/17 Fiona Andrew
5. Eliminating	On walks/garden - normal	Increased frequency of urination	Maintain fluid balance take out frequently	25/3/17 Fiona Andrew
6. Personal cleaning	Hates bathing!	Needs support to clean around vagina ⟷ Dirty around vagina		25/3/17 Fiona Andrew
7. Controlling body temperature	No concerns	Pyrexia	Caused by infection administer pain relief and analgesia	25/3/17 Fiona Andrew
8. Mobilising	Loves walks and chasing balls	Quiet + reluctant to walk	Restricted exercise plan required post-surgery	25/3/17 Fiona Andrew
9. Working and playing	Friendly and enjoys company of people	Quiet unresponsive to voice	Surgical intervention planned	25/3/17 Fiona Andrew
10. Sexuality	Unneutered currently an 'extended' season?	Pyometra	' — ' — '	25/3/17 Fiona Andrew
11. Sleeping	sleeps in dog bed indoors at night	No concerns	Provide bed to get into sleep	25/3/17 Fiona Andrew
12. Dying		Critically ill – but reversible cause, owners aware		25/3/17 Fiona Andrew

Figure 8.6 In practice – Veterinary nursing care plan assessment sheet.

DAILY NURSING CARE PLAN

PATIENT NAME	Dolly
OWNER NAME	W.
BREED	TERRIER
AGE	8 yrs
ADMISSION WEIGHT	6.2 kg
CURRENT WEIGHT	5.8 kg

PRESENTING PROBLEM / DIAGNOSIS _____

MITRAL VALUE DISEASE, CONGESTIVE HEART FAILURE

ALERT VET IF _____ BECOMES SHORT OF BREATH / SIGNS OF DYSPNOEA

OWNER UPDATE CONDITION / COST [✓]   Initials HB

Date 21/3/17

CAN THE PATIENT ?			INITIALS	HB	HB	HB	HB	HB	SR	HB	HB	SR			
		TIME	10^{10}	10^{30}	10^{40}	10^{50}	11^{15}	11^{45}	13^{15}	14^{20}	15^{20}			
BREATHE NORMALLY? MAINTAIN BODY TEMPERATURE ?		RESPIRATORY RATE	52	40	39	39	36	36	32	30				
		O_2 CAGE	✓	✓	✓	✓	✗							
AM NO - NEEDS OXYGEN CAGE	INITIALS HB	HEART RATE	150	140	140	144	130	—	—	124				
		PULSE QUALITY	poor											
AM YES – MONITOR HOURLY	SR	CRT / MM COLOUR	cyanosis	Pink	Pink <2	Pink <2	Pink <2	—	—	Pink				
		TEMPERATURE	38.6	\	\	\	39.2	38.5	—	38.5				
EAT | DRINK		MONITOR GUT SOUNDS	✓	—	—	—	—	—	—					
AM NO DYSPNOEA	HB	FOOD GIVEN (g)	✗	✗	✗	✗	✗	✗	60g	✗				
PM YES	SR	FOOD EATEN (g)	✗	✗	✗	✗	✗	✗	60g	✗				
		WATER in (mL)	200 mL											
URINATE | DEFACATE		URINE OUT BLADDER CHECK ?			✓				✓ out side					
AM YES DIURESIS LIKELY	HB													
PM YES DIURETICS ON GOING	SR	FAECES TYPE							✗					
		VOMIT							✗					
MOBILISE ADEQUATELY + GROOM		WALK / PHYSIO							✓ lead					
AM NO DYSPNOEA	HB	PRESSURE AREA CHECK						✓	✓					
PM YES LEAD WALK ONLY	SR	PAIN P.SCORE						0	0	0				
SLEEP + REST, BEHAVE NORMALLY		DEMEANOUR	Agitated	Dyspnoea			Calmer	Bright	Bright responsive	Wagging Tail calm				
AM MINIMAL HANDLING														
PM ECHO SCAN PLANNED														

MEDICATION	ROUTE	01	02	03	04	05	06	07	08	09	10	11	12	13	14	15	16	17	18	19	20	21	22	23	24
DIUERTIC	IM																								
DIUERTIC	IV										✗														
DIUERTIC	ORAL															✗									

Figure 8.7 Nursing care plan combined with hospitalisation/observation sheet.

DAILY NURSING CARE PLAN

PATIENT NAME _Dolly_	PRESENTING PROBLEM / DIAGNOSIS _____
OWNER NAME _W._	
BREED _TERRIER_	_MITRAL VALUE DISEASE, CONGESTIVE HEART FAILURE_
AGE _8 yrs_	ALERT VET IF _____ _BECOMES SHORT OF BREATH_
ADMISSION _6.2 kg_ CURRENT _5.8 kg_ WEIGHT WEIGHT	_/ SIGNS OF DYSPNOEA_
	OWNER UPDATE CONDITION / COST [✓] Initials _HB_

DATE <u>21/3/17</u>	INDIVIDUALISED NOTES	INITIALS
<u>Time</u> 10^{00}	Admission to ward: discussion with owners Disscussed 1. Diuretic medication / heart scan 2. Explained cyanosis due to lack of O$_2$ 3. Owner asked about prognosis: referred to vet, Dolly not previously on medication so pending results of planned heart scan may be able to start medical management. 4. owner would like to be called any time if changes *CALL MOBILE	HB
11^{15}	Out of O$_2$ cage, dyspnoea resolving, temp high	HB

Figure 8.7 (Continued) Nursing care plan combined with hospitalisation/observation sheet.

However, this may have the disadvantage that it can become a complex document that others not directly involved in the patient's day to day care may struggle to use.

The key point with all the example care plans referred to throughout this textbook is that they are just examples. Each veterinary nursing team should work together to develop their own nursing care plan template to ensure that it is useful and relevant to the clinical practice.

The combined nursing care plan and hospitalisation sheet in Figure 8.7 may not have enough space within it for the sort of polypharmacy that rabbits with gut stasis demand, for example.

That section of the plan should be made larger to accommodate multiple medications in a practice that treats a lot of rabbits. A specialist practice, such as one that works only with patients who have ophthalmology or cardiology conditions, may have a completely different set of observations that must be recorded and they should be reflected in a care plan.

Different models of nursing care may be used, so going back to the specialist ophthalmology practice, using Orem's eight universal needs may facilitate comprehensive patient assessment with enough level of detail to ensure holistic care and allow for the more specialist assessments that are also required. In critical care cases, a more detailed physical approach may be required. Specific critical care assessment models, such as Kirby's Rule of 20 [2], might be used to design a care plan to ensure elements crucial to critically ill patients such as electrolyte imbalance, neurological assessments and coagulation are measured frequently.

Practically, a nursing team might prefer a different format, a landscape format, with fewer tick boxes and more space for subjective commentary. Perhaps one side of the care plan could be used for the day shift and the other side for the night shift care. Different coloured sheets maybe used to identify different vets in charge of individual patients. There is an endless combination of factors reflecting the individual needs of the patient group that a practice is working with. It is only through consideration of those factors can nursing care plans make the transition from tiresome mandated documentation to useful supportive tools for holistic assessment and care.

Review

- The regulatory bodies of both human- and animal-centred nursing provide detailed guidelines for creating and maintaining accurate and useful nursing documentation.
- Goals of care should be set according to SMART principles, which support objective and realistic care goals for the patient.
- Using a predetermined structure of format, such as SOAP, may help nurses construct freehand care plans to cover individualised concepts of patient care.
- Standardised nursing care plans take advantage of the fact that many patients with the same conditions or set of symptoms may require similar interventions. Critical thinking must be applied to ensure that individual patient needs are still taken into account.

Further reflections

Consider the following human-centred clinical situation: imagine you are a nurse in charge of the ward. At 8 am on a surgical recovery ward in the north of England, the surgical consultant is performing a bedside ward round. She greets her first patient, Mrs Jones, and explains to her that she is medically fit for discharge and, if she is happy, she can go home later that day. Mrs Jones is pleased with this news and immediately rings her husband to come and collect her. The conclusion that Mrs Jones is fit for discharge is recorded in the medical notes, signed and dated, and the ward round moves on to the next patient.

At 3 pm you walk through the ward and are surprised to see that Mrs Jones is still on the ward with her husband next to her and her personal property packed at the bottom of the bed. When you enquire as to why Mrs Jones hasn't left yet, she explains that the nurse is looking for somebody to confirm that her central venous catheter may be removed, as she is not allowed home before it is taken out.

When you speak to the nurse looking after Mrs Jones, she explains that although it says in the notes that Mrs Jones is medically fit for discharge, there is no instruction to remove her central venous catheter and the nurse doesn't want to remove it without that explicit instruction and signature.

What do you do?

Take a moment to reflect on this situation and think about the relationship between accurate and contemporary nursing documentation and clinical knowledge and decision-making.

References

1. Royal College of Veterinary Surgeons (2014). Code of Professional Conduct for Veterinary Nurses [online]. Last accessed 28th March 2017. http://www.rcvs.org.uk/advice-and-guidance/code-of-professional-conduct-for-veterinary-nurses/.
2. Kirby R and Linklater A (2016). *Monitoring and Intervention for the Critically Ill Small Animal: The Rule of 20*. Oxford: Wiley.

Further reading

There are many texts available within human-centred nursing that provide examples of nursing care plans that may be adapted to veterinary nursing. There are also examples of resources available that offer guidance on how to appraise information critically in a systematic manner.

1. *Critical Thinking and Writing for Nursing Students*. Bob Price and Anne Harrington (Learning Matters, 2011).
2. *Nursing Care Plans Transitional Patient and Family Centred Care,* 6th edition. Lynda Juall Carpenito (Wolters Kluwer Health, 2014).

Chapter 9

Implementation of nursing care plans

By the end of this chapter you will be able to

1. List barriers to the implementation and effective use of nursing care plans in practice.
2. Appraise the possible explanations for resistance to change within veterinary nursing.
3. Discuss the use of models for managing change.
4. Identify the advantages and disadvantages of using information technology to support care planning.
5. Outline how the TIDE model of implementation of nursing care plans may assist nurses to introduce care planning and care plans to the clinical environment.

The use of nursing care plans has patient-centred advantages as well as having the potential to support professional veterinary practice, as laid out within this textbook. However, there are significant challenges to using nursing care plans in practice. Such challenges may be separated into two categories. First, as the use of nursing care plans is relatively new within veterinary nursing, there are likely to be challenges to the implementation of perceived new practices to a team who may feel they have been working perfectly well without the need for care planning documentation.

Second, there are practical barriers to using care plans. Specifically, there is evidence that veterinary nurses are concerned that care plans take too long to write, are quickly out of date, and can be overly complicated and difficult to understand as different nurses use different abbreviations and terminology.

In human-centred nursing, a report into care planning for patients with long term conditions commissioned by the Department of Health in 2012 [1] provided an interesting insight. The report found that there were so few care plans in place, part of the study was shifted to concentrate on identifying the barriers, perceived and actual, that stopped care plans from being put in place, rather than evaluating their usefulness. The report identified that there was a lack of clarity as to how care plans should be structured, a reluctance to use care plans and an ambivalence concerning the effectiveness and relevance of nursing care plans.

Resistance to change

Change and adaption of practice is an essential part of adhering to the nursing code of conduct, both in veterinary and human-centred nursing. Both codes of conduct mandate clinical governance and using care that is based on the best possible evidence. The implication therefore is that, as evidence for care changes, so must the care that is administered change. These principles of clinical governance are only as good as the implementation of change in practice.

Clinical governance strategy that identifies the need for change but has no mechanism to implement it has no place in healthcare.

There are many reasons as to why nursing staff in particular may be resistant to change in practice. Historically, both nursing professions have held a subordinate role, under the direct instruction of a doctor or veterinary surgeon. It is this background that may make nursing staff wary of suggesting change in practice, or implementing different ways of working.

Other traditional and ritualistic features of nursing may lead to a negative reaction to implementing change in practice. Nursing has a long history of being taught via word of mouth, with senior staff passing on their experiences and knowledge to juniors. This form of teaching does not encourage a depth of understanding about the subject being discussed. Information exchange is likely to be functional, practical, with little explanation of theory or why the intervention is being carried out. Therefore, it may lead to nursing staff who are confident within their remit of work, however, resistant to change due to a lack of comprehension as to why they are performing the care they do. For example, a student nurse may have been taught how to prepare intravenous fluid therapy for an animal. Traditionally, they may have been taught which fluid should be given to which particular disease process, or set of symptoms. However, what happens when the relevant fluid is out of stock, or an animal presents with symptoms that overlap and may indicate two different types of fluids? The nurse is unable to think laterally and decide which fluid is appropriate, because they have no knowledge of what each fluid consists of and what each fluid is doing for the patient. Steps have been taken to address this issue, and since 2006, veterinary nursing students are taught differently so that critical thinking and application of practice is encouraged. There are still nurses who apply this method of teaching and it is those nurses and their pupils who may struggle with changes to established practice and therefore be resistant to implementing them.

As has been mentioned within this text, there is a limited amount of evidence-based resources available to guide clinical veterinary nursing practice. This has led to care interventions that have been based on tradition, ritual and anecdotal evidence. These may be long-standing and therefore, again, difficult to replace with new care strategies.

A combination of these factors may lead to the idea of changes to practice being very stressful for nursing staff. This, in itself, is a barrier to change as nurses who are fearful of change are less likely to implement it and even less likely to advocate for it.

In 2013, Wager and Welsh [2] investigated the experiences of 56 registered veterinary nurses implementing a framework for planning care within practice, specifically, using Orpet and Jeffery's Ability Model of care. They documented a clear negative emotional response experienced by the veterinary nurse when given the task of implementing documented care planning in their practice. They described feeling apprehensive, nervous, stressed, worried, fearful and anxious. This outlines one of the key challenges that anyone who advocates care planning will meet almost immediately. There seems to be a perception within the veterinary nursing profession that planning care is something to be anxious or frightened of. In fact, it is something that is done every day, often all day. Implicitly, veterinary nurses are constantly assessing patients, checking they have everything they need, and advising their colleagues on what they have done so that the care can be continued throughout the day and night.

In veterinary nursing, resistance to a change of practice surrounding nursing care plans may be compounded by the fact that many veterinary nurses in practice may not have received any education about nursing care plans during their training. There is a strong chance that the veterinary nurse who is advocating the use of nursing care plans may be relatively newly qualified and therefore have received training on the benefits of planning care and using nursing care plans during their nursing education. This may augment a primitive resistance to implementation of nursing care plans as more experienced nurses resent the idea that they require a care plan to assist them to care for their patients.

Reasons why nurses may resist change in practice

- Historical – subordinate role/education
- Reluctance to learn from less experienced members of the team
- Practice based on tradition and ritual
- Source of stress
- Lack of time

An introduction to implementation of change models

Consideration of these potential barriers to change must be taken into account when any new practice is suggested. Change that is enforced on staff, without agreement and engagement, can lead to increased staff turnover, hostility in the work place, low morale and a stronger resistance to any further change.

There are several models for implementing change available and one of the most familiar is Lewin's work from the 1950s [3]. This consists of a three-stage process: unfreezing, changing and refreezing.

Unfreezing is essentially an information-gathering stage; at this point, those wishing to implement change in practice are encouraged to gather a clear understanding of the current situation and identify the problems that need addressing with change. This should incorporate consideration of the views of key stakeholders, resource availability, and identification of personnel so that a team may be put together to lead the change and support and guide other members of staff. Finally, it will involve putting a detailed plan together for how the change may be implemented, taking care to ensure that clear lines of communication are prioritised to inform and support team members.

The **changing** stage is the implementation of change and primarily consists of the training and updating of stakeholders. Clear communication is essential when trying to implement a change in practice. The expectations of the team need to be clear and the goals of the change must be widely disseminated. Staff need to understand the principles behind the need for change and the potential benefits that the change may have to patients and or staff.

Finally, Lewin advocates a stage of **refreezing**. At this point, the change in practice is evaluated and if it has achieved its aims, it may be ingrained into the normal working day. Here, again, communication is key. All staff must be kept up to date as to the progress of the change, they must know if it is to go ahead, or staff maybe confused and disheartened and return to traditional practice while some continue with the new practice. This may result in poor patient outcomes as different staff members end up with different goals of care for the same patient.

A second model of change widely used within the NHS is the PDSA cycle. Originally constructed by Edward Demming in the 1950s [4], it remains a useful tool to implement and evaluate change in practice. It is a four-stage cyclical process which advocates a considered and structured plan: do, study, act, approach. It puts a priority on defining clear objectives, identifying the change that is required, and ensuring that changes to practice are evaluated and, if necessary, put through a second change cycle to ensure they are robust and relevant to practice. The key advantage of the PDSA cycle is the clear language and terminology which is relatively self-explanatory and therefore makes this an accessible and useful model of change (Figure 9.1).

A third model of change, the Appreciative Leadership approach (AL) moves the focus of implementation of change away from problem solving and concentrates on identifying good practice and establishing how that good practice may be improved. Originally described by Cooperrider and Srivasta in 1987 [5], it prioritises staff involvement. It aims to avoid the potential conflict associated with other models that concentrate on implementing change based on the identification of a problem or issue of poor care. This may lead to low staff morale and disengagement if staff believe they are being blamed for past failures and are not part of any potential solution to issues.

AL should be implemented as a four-stage process. The discovery phase, which consists of appreciative inquiry, is the core of the model. It involves asking questions to establish what staff believe is good about their practice and how they feel it might be improved. Next, the dream phase asks staff how practice may be improved. Following that, staff are asked to contribute ideas about a united vision for their role, ward, or department. Finally, they are asked how they may go about achieving their vision. This may incorporate both physical resources and emotional input to assist changes in attitude. The caveat to such a process is the need for demonstrable and measurable action after the engaging with staff. AL may quickly lead to low morale and disengagement if it is used within a system that cannot provide resource and change in response to staff ideas. Careful management is required to ensure staff are listened to and any appropriate and relevant solutions they have suggested are carried out and followed through.

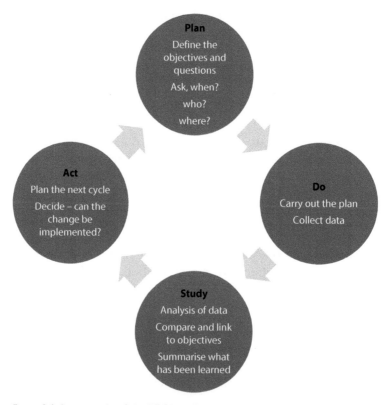

Figure 9.1 **An example of the PDSA cycle.**

Conversely, careful explanation is required should plans and ideas not be useful or possible so staff understand why their input has not been taken up.

Thinking critically about nursing care plans

There are three main barriers to the practical use of nursing care plans which may be considered significant disadvantages of the practical use nursing care plans. Alongside the marked negative emotional responses to the implementation of nursing care plans, Wagner and Welsh's study (2013) revealed that one of the most frequent observations made by the veterinary nurses in the study was that planning care was too time-consuming. This observation supported a similar conclusion from Brown in 2012 [6]. The concerns around timing led many of the veterinary nurses questioned to state that they felt care planning was not practical. There was a sense that patient care may be neglected in order to complete the patient documentation.

Barriers to the use of nursing care plans in practice

1. Writing care plans takes too long.
2. Terminology is confusing and means time is wasted establishing what care plans mean.
3. Care plan rapidly becomes out of date so it is useless minutes after it is written.

Second, in both human and veterinary centred nursing there are regular concerns voiced about keeping care plans relevant as patient needs change. In an interesting editorial, La Duke [7] argues that nursing care plans are actually a hindrance to nurses rather than an adjuvant. Her theory is that nurses continually receive and analyse new data about their patient and, most importantly, have to act on that data. The need for constant manual revision of a care plan may keep the nurse from fulfilling care needs.

Third, in 2012, Brown highlighted an important criticism of using a formal written care plans in practice, the use of abbreviations and medical terminology. She observed that a significant amount of time was spent writing detailed explanations on a care plan to ensure that all colleagues would be able to understand and engage with the patient care. If terminology is poorly understood and personalised abbreviations used without consideration as to who understands them, team members may struggle to understand the plan of care. Knowledge of terminology and abbreviations is influenced by a number of factors including culture, heritage, and education. While working in Australia, the author recalls comparing the size of a dog's bladder to that of a satsuma. A note was left for the surgeon to that effect, in an attempt at reassurance. The surgeon, confused and bewildered, sent an amusing message asking, 'What on earth is a satsuma?!' In this case, clearly a scale of size based on fruit was not appropriate!

Consideration of the amount of time assigned to care planning and associated nursing documentation highlights one subject where the veterinary nursing profession may learn from their human-centred counterparts. The perception of there being too much paperwork within human nursing is well-documented. Indeed, while working within the NHS, the author has experienced the dilemma of knowing there is only the time before the end of a shift to either perform the care required, or document the fact that there is no time to perform the care required. There is not actually the time to both do the care and document it appropriately. It is this sort of dilemma that when it occurs every day, might lead to care being missed, documentation not being kept up to date, or nurses working unpaid overtime to ensure that their patients receive appropriate care.

Such situations are seldom solely due to paperwork, and healthcare within the UK is a uniquely complex situation. However, the use of overly complicated and repetitive paperwork is a problem. In one department, the author recalls taking the blood pressure of a patient, which then had to be written down on four individual sheets of paper. One sheet was to go to the consultant, who was due to see the patient. A second sheet stayed in the nursing notes to facilitate examination of trends and anomalies. A third sheet went to the medical secretaries and data team who, later that day, would write up the consultant's letter about the patient; and the fourth went with the patient to the diagnostics department to be used as part of their pre-procedure assessment. It was indeed a long and laborious process. A further anecdote from a mental health nurse who recalls that during an admission of a patient, he wrote the patient's weight and height on seven individual pieces of paper.

In using time-consuming, complicated, and repetitive paperwork to support care planning, the real dangers are that care plans and nursing models will be adapted by nurses keen to save time, and aspects of the model that are deemed irrelevant will be ignored. Alternatively, the care plan may be omitted altogether in patients who are not deemed to be staying in the veterinary hospital long enough to justify the care planning process. This would be unfortunate, as in a 24-hour period an animal still needs to eat, drink and groom itself. So, if the relevant assessment information has been recorded on a care plan, care can be implemented and potential problems avoided. So, a dog that has been hit by a car now has a repaired fracture and adequate pain relief, but refuses his food. Upon referring to a comprehensive care plan, the nurse looking after him can see his favourite food is freshly cooked chicken, fetches some out of the freezer and gets it cooked, where upon the dog duly eats it. This means he maintains his nutritional status, which then has a positive impact on his electrolyte, albumin, calorific and hydration status, potentially avoiding further interventions such as intravenous fluid therapy or assisted nutrition.

The same principles apply in human-centred nursing. When treating a person with a heart attack, is it really necessary to assess his sleep pattern in the previous few weeks leading up to the event? Possibly not in that acutely unwell moment, but later on, yes. Consider if on asking that patient how their sleep is, they reply that they struggle to sleep; intense stress from work is keeping them awake plus they often have to sleep almost sitting up, as lying down leaves them short of breath. These are clear and relevant factors that may impact the patient's ongoing care; the first indicates the need to address their lifestyle and the second may indicate a more chronic heart problem.

Knowing the home environment of an elderly patient when they are admitted with a fractured hip may not feel relevant as they are transferred to surgery to have their hip repaired. However, such information becomes essential when planning for discharge and suddenly the team realise that the patient lives in a third-floor flat in a building with an unreliable lift.

The counter argument to those who would like to save time and eliminate and adapt parts of a nursing model is clear: we don't know what we don't know. Potentially, an interaction with a healthcare professional could be a step out of an abusive relationship, the resolve of a difficult painful ongoing set of symptoms or an opportunity to improve an unhealthy lifestyle. These opportunities might well be missed, should a thorough assessment be missed. The key point is that a model such as RLT, Orem and the Ability Model have been developed to ensure that nothing is missed and that care remains focused to the full set of needs of the patient.

Implementing nursing care plans into practice

There may be significant challenges to overcome when nurses set out to try and introduce nursing care plans to practice. The potential disadvantages to using a nursing care plan that is long and cumbersome are clear, and resistance to change is a perfectly natural phenomenon in teams of staff that have been working in a particular way for some time.

TIDE stands for training, information technology, design, and evaluation, and is a simple acronym specifically written to provide a reminder of four key points that should be considered when introducing nursing care plans to veterinary practice.

Implementation of nursing care plans

Think **TIDE** – training, information technology, design and evaluation.

Training

The importance of training and education is demonstrated by the well-established models of implementing change. Within the context of veterinary nursing, if nurses do not understand the function or the potential benefits of using nursing care plans they may be ambivalent to their use or worse, feel stressed, anxious and concerned about using nursing care plans. Concepts such as models of care and the veterinary nursing process may be dismissed as complex, abstract ideas, rejected in favour of simply getting on with the job. The idea that all patients, animal or human, should be offered care plans to optimise their care is only useful if there is clear support and training for all staff involved. Without it, care plans are likely to be a purely cosmetic exercise, with little to no practical use at all.

Training may manifest in a range of ways, from online training, attendance of continuing professional development meetings such as British Association of Veterinary Nurses congress, in-house training from senior staff members through formal presentations, or external accredited qualifications.

Within the NHS, training staff about changes in clinical practice is often coordinated by link nurses. Link nurses are staff members who have identified a specific area of nursing that they are interested in. They take on the responsibility of ensuring they attend training sessions and liaise with specialists to learn about current best practice and policy so they may disseminate it among their frontline nursing colleagues. As a typical example, most ward teams throughout the NHS will have an infection control link nurse. They become the named contact on the ward should there be any need for updates on clinical practice regarding infection control issues. Such updates may include the need to isolate patients with certain identified infections, or the dissemination of risk assessment documents to establish the likelihood of infections. Additionally, many link nurses are responsible for conducting audits within their area of interest to ensure the principles of clinical governance are being applied and care is being measured. Link nurses often become excellent advocates for establishing high standards of practice within their area of interest. Peer to peer learning can be a productive form of training, seeing others engaged with particular methods or applications of practice may mean that colleagues of link nurses are far more likely to adapt their practice and implement change.

Potentially, there are many professional benefits for staff, should they volunteer for such a role. Their development of specialist knowledge may increase their professional satisfaction as they feel empowered to support their colleagues in teaching and guiding their practice to facilitate better outcomes for patients. Link nurse roles offer the opportunity to attend senior staff meetings as their role incorporates the dissemination of information that is discussed at such meetings. It may also offer the opportunity to develop skills in clinical audit management and presentation of information.

The link nurse model is one that may easily be applied to veterinary nursing. Implementing a new practice or a change is easier if there are multiple members of the team engaged in the process and willing to share their knowledge and enthusiasm with others. Link nurses within the NHS may hold roles linked with health and safety, nursing documentation, and information technology, as well as more clinical aspects of care such as diabetes, delirium, stroke, and dementia. It is reasonable to suggest that veterinary practice might also benefit from the development of link nurses in such areas as wound management, infection control, zoonosis and nursing care planning.

Information technology

Technology is used widely in human-centred healthcare. From the high-tech engineering used to develop mobility aids, the use of robotic technology for minimally invasive surgery, renal dialysis machines, imaging and diagnostics; it is everywhere. And yet, step into most wards towards the end of a shift and there will be many nurses, sitting at desks, separate from the patients, with heads bent and biros in hand writing out the day's events.

Recording the events of an 8- to 12-hour shift in the last 20 minutes of that relentlessly busy shift cannot be the best way of keeping a record of what has happened, evaluating the care plans or developing a new care plan to hand over to the new staff. Consulting guidelines for constructing nursing documentation is clear that all documentation should be contemporaneous. It may be argued that writing up events that happened at 7:20 am at 5:20 pm is not a contemporary record; it is easy for details to be forgotten and key elements of care not recorded.

Nursing is becoming busier and busier with higher patient morbidity and shorter lengths of patient stay contributing to a faster turnover of patients and to a larger workload day to day. In addition, the same factors emphasise the importance of clear and relevant care planning and documentation. Complex patients with significant co-morbidities require holistic assessment to ensure that all their needs are being met. Development of tools to support efficient care planning and documentation are essential to support nursing care.

The obvious solution is to develop technological solutions. While computerised requests for diagnostics, referrals, and supplies are commonplace in many hospitals, computerised nursing care plans are much less common. However, there are many time-saving opportunities that may be created using computerised nursing care plans.

Advantages of computerised nursing care plans

Computerised care plans are generally quick and easy to fill in, pre-population of entries may be facilitated, and nurses simply need to click and drag the relevant entry. Such easy access encourages documentation at the time of treatment or intervention, instead of writing everything at the end of a shift. Comprehensive online care plans may reduce the need for comment and narrative; they can streamline the information recorded which saves time. There will be immediate access to the entire history of the patient care within that stay, and potentially, previous stays, plus the ability to swiftly search entries to identify trends and changes. Referrals may be automated, triggers can be set to alert other members of specialist staff if particular changes occur in the patient's condition. The referral process will be quicker as notes can be accessed remotely by other members of the multidisciplinary team, or emailed at the press of a button, saving the need for a written narrative of a complex and lengthy admission.

Alongside the potential time-saving element of using computerised nursing care plans, such systems are designed specifically to fulfil professional guidelines for effective documentation.

So, a computerised system will facilitate clear recognition of the patient to which it applies to. Log in systems, protected by passwords, ensure it is clear who is entering the data and when that data is entered. Entries onto such a system become a permanent and legible record of care, with less likelihood of omissions through lost pieces of paper. Errors that may have previously occurred due to illegible handwriting are now avoided and the potential for ambiguity may be greatly decreased. Confidential data may be better protected through the use of password protected systems as opposed to folders of care plans lying around the ward. They may be used as a learning tool, programmes may be set up so that once a particular nursing diagnosis is entered, relevant interventions automatically flag up. Also, pop-ups and reminders may be set to ensure that mandatory assessments are performed regularly. Pressure area care or nutrition are obvious subjects, and directing a nurse's attention to them is likely to remind them they need addressing, working towards a holistic approach. Professionally, the use of computerised nursing care plans provides the opportunity for nurses to develop IT skills on a day to day basis. Additionally, these computerised systems may become huge repositories of data which might be utilised for research, policy, commissioning decisions or management of the service. Finally, there may be environmental and cost-saving benefits as less printing is carried out and therefore, less paper is used.

Advantages of computerised nursing care plans

Time-saving advantages
- Quicker to complete
- Immediate access to entire history of patient care
- Automated referrals
- Efficient communication between MDT members through email
- Streamlining of information
- Facilitation of contemporary records

Other benefits
- Provides a permanent and legible record of care
- Password protected entries record time and person entering data
- Reduction in errors associated with lost records or illegible handwriting
- Source of data
- Support for holistic care
- Learning tool
- Development of new IT skills
- Improved patient confidentiality
- Environmental benefits

Disadvantages of computerised nursing care plans

While there are many potential advantages of using computerised nursing care plans there are significant disadvantages and barriers to the implementation of such a system.

First, there is potentially a huge capital outlay and the need to address the equally large logistical factors of facilitating computerised recording of care within a healthcare environment.

Additionally, the fact that such equipment is going into a healthcare environment may result in the need for the use of specialised materials such as water resistant, easy-to-clean keyboards which can increase the cost of implementation significantly, perhaps restrictively. Furthermore, systems will need to be put in place to ensure that systems are secure, confidential patient information is protected, and support is available should there be a malfunction. Such services require ongoing financial input.

Professionally, not all nursing staff may be confident in working with computers and therefore, supportive measures, training, and education will need to be implemented. Systems of peer support, and the opportunity to practice populating patient records within a supportive environment need to be implemented. While this might be an opportunity to develop new skills and learn, not all members of staff are likely to see it that way. Such methods in practice might be a huge source of concern and anxiety for those not familiar with computers. Equally, on a busy, overstretched hospital or veterinary practice, it may be difficult to release staff to complete the relevant training.

Multidisciplinary working

There is also an argument that such computerised systems could restrict conversations between MDT members, which may stifle collaborative practice and the development of new ideas for practice. Reliance on automated referrals and email communication may negate the need for healthcare practitioners to see the patient together and therefore prevent face to face communication and debrief about the individual's care. Such face to face interaction often has an informal advantage of implicit support and reflection as cases are shared and opinions sought from senior, more experienced colleagues.

While one of the advantages of using such a system may be increased patient confidentiality, conversely, without diligent attention to principles of **information governance**, the structures, policies and procedures put into place to protect data, such as not sharing passwords, ensuring all terminals are logged out of information, may be vulnerable to inappropriate sharing.

Patient-centred care

A record that involves filling in a template, also runs the risk of lacking a patient-centred approach. A patient's unique, individual needs may not be recorded if they are not part of a recognised approach to that set of symptoms or care needs. It is difficult to think of all the possible outcomes for an assessment and therefore it is likely that nurses may find themselves unable to find a box to put their particular patient-specific entry in. This may lead them to omit such an entry believing it to be superfluous, resulting in a poorer patient experience. Consider a person who is a patient in a hospital and has a phobia of needles. This is a significant issue, and is likely to be a significant issue throughout their stay in hospital regardless of the ward they are on. As an added complication, there is a need for many members of the multidisciplinary team to know and understand their phobia so that care may be designed to support the patient. Nursing notes that are kept specifically on a computer may result in staff members not knowing about such an important issue. Junior doctors are often responsible for intravenous access and phlebotomy but may not necessarily access nursing notes. Phlebotomists, consultants and nursing assistants all need to know, but, again, may not access nursing notes on a computer system. However, in contrast, a care plan at the end of a bed can be easily accessed.

Completing a template on the computer may be an efficient way of documenting care, as it negates the need for nurses to spend time constructing a detailed narrative account of the care that has been given. While this is beneficial, it must be remembered that there is a need for nurses to retain some skills in narrative record keeping. Computer templates and tick boxes cannot account for the documentation of all patient details. An example is the need to document communication with both the patient and their relatives. Guidance from both the human-centred and veterinary nursing regulatory bodies mandate the information given to the patient and their support network must be documented. This relies on accurate and detailed record-keeping from the nurse.

Disadvantages of computerised nursing care plans

- Costs
- Education and training
- Restriction of MDT conversations
- Reduction in patient-centred approach to care
- Loss of narrative writing skills
- Information governance violation

Design

The third element of TIDE stands for design. The inclusion of this word is to remind nursing staff that nursing care plans may be designed specifically for the practice in which they will be used. Several example care plans are given in chapter eight with the caveat that they are simply examples. Before trying to use a care plan in practice, it is essential that all relevant stakeholders, so anyone who has an interest or concern in using nursing plans, has an opportunity to put their views across. As an example, a manager might be battling with debt control and so, wants to highlight the need for a section on the care plan to remind staff to update owners on the cumulative cost of their animal's treatment. The nursing team, aware of a varying level of experience within their team might suggest specific assessment tools are used in conjunction with the care plan to try and minimise the subjective variation in terminology and abbreviations. Veterinary surgeons keen to ensure they are kept up to date with any changes to the patient's condition might advocate for inclusion of a section they can edit with triggers for alerting them.

Consultations with staff ensure nursing care plans are implemented with consideration of the context of their use. It is understandable that an experienced veterinary nurse, unfamiliar with the use of nursing care plans, might feel a little affronted to have a new tool inflicted on them. They may feel that their existing nursing skills and experience are being questioned or disregarded. This is not the case; in fact, experienced nurses should be encouraged to use nursing care plans in different ways. Experienced nurses are likely to be planning care implicitly and therefore may find completing nursing care plans tiresome. Experienced nurses may be able to use a nursing care plan as a simple aide memoir to support their practice. It may provide them with a tool to support and teach less experienced nurses. It might also stimulate research questions, or audit opportunities, so that they may improve their practice and improve the care their patients receive. Furthermore, it is likely that the experienced nurses may be the ones who develop nursing care plans for home care when supporting the owners of chronically ill animals.

In contrast, a nursing care plan may be an excellent tool to support newly qualified nurses. It can provide direction of care and stimulate a new nurse to seek out the advice and support of an experienced colleague should they reach a stage in the nursing of a patient that they are unable to facilitate unaided.

Evaluation

Finally, E stands for evaluation. Evaluation of any applied change in practice is essential. The importance of evaluation is demonstrated when considering the clinical audit cycle; once a change in practice has been implemented, there is need for further evaluation and assessment to check that the change in practice is actually useful and achieving what it was supposed to do. The same applies when developing nursing care plans for a practice previously not using them. Once the time is right, the care plan may be used by clinical staff; however, it is sensible to set a date where further consultation may be sought with colleagues to ensure it is indeed fulfilling its objectives.

Using a framework to structure the process of care might be relatively new to the veterinary nursing profession, but it shouldn't be difficult and certainly shouldn't be frightening or stressful. Writing care plans can take time, but it may be argued that it is time well spent. A detailed and contemporary nursing care plan fulfils multiple functions. It may provide a global overview of care needs, stimulate evaluation of care, manage risk to patients through consideration of potential problems as well as actual ones, and can be used as an education tool. All nurses involved need to understand the function and benefits of such a care plan or there is a danger of the care planning process becoming more of a hindrance than a help.

Review

- The use of nursing care plans may be challenged; nurses may believe they are too time consuming and be reluctant to change their current practice.
- Specific models of working exist to support the implementation of change.
- Clear communication is one of the most important tools when seeking to implement a change in practice.
- Nursing is becoming increasingly busy; nurses should seek out and test tools to support efficient and effective documentation, including the use of information technology when appropriate.

Further reflections

One of the biggest changes within the workplace is a change in colleagues, as existing staff leave for different opportunities and new staff are employed to replace them. Use a change model, perhaps one of the examples in this chapter, and apply it to supporting the introduction of a new staff member to the team. Incorporate the needs of both the new staff member and the existing team. Think about which strategies are already in place for such an eventuality and how they may be extended or improved. Consider both the clinical and the non-clinical angles of their future role and the support that may be offered.

References

1. Department of Health (2012). Care Planning in the Treatment of Long Term Conditions a Final Report of the CAPITOL Project [online]. Last accessed 28th March 2017. http://hrep .lshtm.ac.uk/publications/Care%20planning_final_Bower%20et%20al_7%20Mar%2013.pdf.
2. Welsh P and Wager C (2013). Veterinary nurses creating a unique approach to patient care: Part one. *The Veterinary Nurse*, 4 (8), 452–459.
3. Lewin K (1947). Frontiers in group dynamics: Concept, method and reality in social science: Social equilibria and social change. *Human Relations*, 1, 1, 5–41.
4. Institue of Healthcare Improvement (2017). The PDSA Cycle [online]. Last accessed 29th March 2017. http://www.ihi.org/resources/Pages/HowtoImprove/ScienceofImprovement ImplementingChanges.aspx.
5. Cooperrider D and Srivastva S (1987). Appreciative inquiry in organisational life. Research in organisational change and development. In Woodman R and Pasmore W (Eds.), *Research in Organisational Change and Development*. Volume 1. Greenwich CT: JAI Press.
6. Brown C (2012). Experience of designing and implementing a care plan in the veterinary environment. *The Veterinary Nurse*, 3 (9), 534–542.
7. LaDuke S (2008). Death to nursing care plans! *American Journal of Nursing*, 108, 6, 13.

Further reading

Managing change with health is a key aspect of healthcare leadership; these resources offer further ideas on developing a unique change strategy.

1. *Practical Leadership in Nursing and Health Care – A Multi-Professional Approach*. Suzanne Henwood (CRC Press, 2014).
2. *Leadership in Health and Social Care*. Louise Jones and Clare Bennett (Lantern Publishing, 2012).
3. *ABC of Clinical Leadership*. Tim Swanwick and Judy McKimm (Wiley Blackwell, 2011).

Chapter 10

The future of nursing care plans in veterinary nursing

By the end of this chapter you will be able to

1. Discuss the reasons human-centred nurses have developed additional care planning tools.
2. Define and differentiate between nursing care plans, care bundles and integrated care pathways.
3. Identify the stages of writing a care bundle and apply them to writing a care bundle for veterinary nursing.
4. Propose examples of how veterinary nursing care may be improved by the use of a care planning tool.
5. Speculate on how novel tools for care planning may be applied to veterinary nursing in the future.

Nursing care plans are used widely throughout human-centred nursing, however, there have been questions asked surrounding their use. There are significant barriers to the use of nursing care plans in practice, specifically, the length of time it can take to complete the plan and the possibility of it quickly becoming out of date. Human-centred nursing has developed strategies to combat these barriers. Subsequently, these strategies, some say, have now made the care plan redundant. In a world of national care guidelines and information technology, nurses are asking if their care plans are really relevant and necessary to provide patient-centred care.

Within the NHS, alongside the recognised limitations of using nursing care plans, there are other factors and pressures that have led to the development of tools to support the planning of patient care. Increased multi-disciplinary input into patients who have increasingly complex needs has led to the development of documentation tools and programmes that focus on recording nursing input alongside and in conjunction with the input of other team members. Increasingly complex discharge planning and the pressure to discharge patients due to bed shortages have meant that nurses may increasingly find themselves in the role of care coordinator as they facilitate home support, carer education and patient transfers. This has led to an emphasis on documentation that supports early discharge planning so that elements of discharge such as transportation requirements, home care and financial assessments may be identified in advance to facilitate a smooth discharge process. The need for effective resource management in an NHS that is financially overstretched has emphasised the need to develop tools that support the use of robust evidence-based practice where possible.

Given that veterinary nursing has a history of echoing developments in human-centred nursing, it is likely that some of these issues may well affect the veterinary profession in due course. Certainly the call for evidenced-based practice is already underway in veterinary nursing. Just like people, animals are living longer and longer, with more complex needs. Plus, in an ever-changing financial situation, owners may have less spare money to spend on veterinary treatment and therefore, careful resource management may become more and more relevant. Applying the principles of clinical governance, it is sensible to look to human-centred nursing and ask whether any tools currently in use may facilitate a more effective care model for animals.

Care bundles

One such tool is the care bundle. A care bundle is defined as a group of evidence-based practices related to a disease or set of symptoms that, when executed together, result in better outcomes than when implemented individually [1]. The evidence used to develop care bundles reflects strong science, usually involving at least one systematic review of multiple, well designed, randomised controlled trials. Clinically, the use of care bundles has been credited with improved patient outcomes in a number of disease processes or sets of symptoms. A successful example is the implementation of ventilator care bundles. In 2012, the Institute for Healthcare Improvement [2] developed an evidence-based list of interventions that were linked to reductions in ventilator-associated pneumonia in ventilated patients in the ICU. These included positioning of the head, regular assessment for extubation, oral care and daily sedation breaks (Figure 10.1).

As a result, clear benefits have been seen; hundreds of hospitals employing ventilator care bundles have now experienced several years without any cases of ventilator-acquired pneumonia [3].

The treatment of sepsis is a second well documented example. Sepsis is a known or suspected infection with a systemic manifestation of infection and is associated with high mortality rates in human patients across the UK. The first sepsis care bundle was published in 2004 and has been subsequently updated based on the practice guidelines published by the Surviving Sepsis Campaign [4].

A commonly used adaptation of the bundle guidelines used across the UK is the Sepsis six (Figure 10.2). This is a list of six key interventions that can be performed once a patient begins

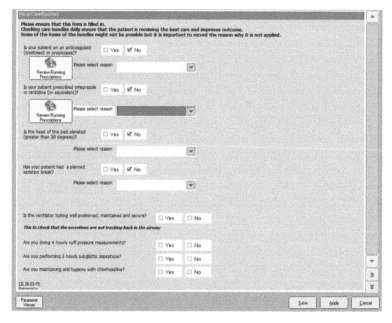

Figure 10.1 **Human-centred ventilator care bundle. (Reproduced from Papworth Hospital NHS Foundation Trust. With kind permission.)**

suffering symptoms indicating that they may be septic. The interventions include: administration of high-flow oxygen (to maintain target oxygen saturations), administration of intravenous fluids, obtaining blood cultures, measurement of lactate, administration of intra venous antibiotics, and measurement of fluid output.

Each of these interventions is important either in treating infection or monitoring the impact of the treatment of infection. From a nursing point of view, several of these interventions can be implemented autonomously while escalating concerns to the medical team. So, a fluid chart can be started to monitor urine output, an existing intra venous line can be flushed and prepared or a new one placed, blood samples can be taken, and equipment can be prepared.

In 2010, a detailed analysis of the results of the Surviving Sepsis Campaign and associated care bundles indicated a reduction in mortality from 37% to 30.8% over a two-year period [5]. In 2012, The Institute of Healthcare Improvement published a White Paper titled 'Using care bundles to improve healthcare quality' [5]. The authors describe care bundles as a ground-breaking strategy to improve patient care outcomes through use of best practices and innovation.

There is further evidence that care bundles used to manage exacerbations in chronically ill patients have also improved clinical outcomes. They have supported patients to manage their condition more effectively, and promote a standardised evidence-based approach. It may be surmised that the improvement in patient outcomes is due to the fact that evidence-based interventions are being used. While this is relevant, it is too simplistic a view. Care bundles support efficient and effective teamworking; initiation of a care bundle directs a team to work in a knowledgeable and

DN598 - Management of SIRS / Sepsis Guideline

Papworth Hospital NHS
NHS Foundation Trust

Papworth Hospital NHS
NHS Foundation Trust

Addressograph
Name:
Date of birth:
Hosp No:
NHS No:

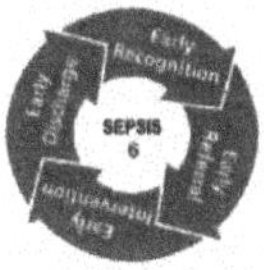

Ensure doctor and ALERT attend NOW and work together to achieve these tasks

Sepsis 6 Care Bundle Date Commenced: Ward Area:

	Complete within 1 hour	Time	Initial	Result	Reason not done and rationale
Investigations	**1. Take blood cultures** Perform septic screen i.e. urine, sputum, swabs, lines. Consider also imaging to find source i.e. CXR - ideally all prior to commencing antibiotics (If vascular access device in situ take cultures both peripherally and via device)				
	2. Measure lactate (ABG/routine bloods with CRP) If >2mmol/l: give up to 10ml/kg Hartmann's or 0.9% saline (unless already given)				
	3. Measure accurate urine output May need catheterising, start fluid balance chart				
Treatments	**4. Give a fluid challenge** If Syst BP< 90: STAT up to 10ml/kg Hartmann's or 0.9% saline (alternatively use a colloid) *Note: LV function/pulmonary oedema*				
	5. Give IV antibiotics According to Trust protocol (available on intranet) within 1hr and following blood cultures				
	6. Give high-flow oxygen Reservoir mask at 15 litres unless COPD.(If COPD administer oxygen to maintain patients oxygen saturations within target range as per Trust Guidelines.)				

	Complete within 6 hours	Time	Initial	Result	Reason not done and rationale
Ongoing	**1. Re measure Lactate** if initial result elevated				
	2. Measure Blood Pressure if persistent hypotension				
	3. Consider Referral to CCA if appropriate (i.e. persistent hypotension)				

CN 177 Sepsis Bundle Paperwork File Section: 2

CN177 Sepsis Bundle: Section 2

Figure 10.2 The Sepsis six care bundle. (Reproduced from Papworth Hospital NHS Foundation Trust. With kind permission.)

effective manner. Team members have clear shared goals and tasks may be matched up to the relevant staff members and implemented swiftly. Responsibility for completing the bundle can be shared across the team contributing to a sense of cohesion and collaborative practice.

A completed care bundle, as a stand-alone document, provides evidence of the interventions that have been performed for an individual patient. Collectively, they may provide the basis of a useful audit. Once a care bundle is put in place, it is prudent to examine the paperwork and establish that all the relevant interventions are carried out. Returning to the sepsis bundle, one of the clear instructions is that blood culture samples should be taken before intra venous antibiotics are given. On examination of a series of sepsis care bundles, it may be noted that the one intervention that is not completed 100% of the time is in fact the venepuncture for obtaining blood culture samples. If so, measures may be implemented to understand why this stage in the process is proving difficult. Nurses might describe not feeling adequately skilled to take blood culture samples or are struggling to find the necessary equipment. The care bundle audit will provide evidence so that funding may be obtained for further venepuncture training or for the sourcing and relocation of the relevant resources.

Benefits of using care bundles

- Improve patient outcomes
- Reduced gap between theory and practice
- Measurable record of care
- Increased team working
- Time saving

Writing a care bundle

There are five clear stages to writing a care bundle. The first stage involves selecting a specific care theme. The second stage is to identify a cluster of interventions or practices that are associated with that theme. The third stage is to perform a literature search on the interventions to try and establish what evidence there is for their use. The fourth stage of writing a care bundle involves the categorisation of the evidence associated with a particular intervention according to its quality. This involves the application of critical thinking to the problem, alongside robust consultation with stakeholders. It is generally accepted that the highest level research involves the use of evidence from at least one systematic review, or meta-analysis, of well-designed randomised controlled trials (RCTs) or evidence from at least one RCT of appropriate size. Interventions associated with strong evidence may be used as part of the care bundle. The fifth and final step of writing a care bundle is to delete any interventions that do not have robust evidence associated with them.

Care bundles rely on the use of evidence-based practice. There is a well-known gap between the theory of nursing and medicine and the practice that occurs day to day. There can be a long journey between the laboratory and the bedside or kennel in a veterinary hospital. This may be due to a number of factors. In veterinary nursing, it is most likely due to the difficulties in accessing evidence-based information and potential restrictions placed on implementing such measures due to financial constraints. Similar restrictions occur within human-centred medicine, specifically, it may be difficult for nurses to access contemporary high quality evidence about their practice. Care bundles address that gap. The interventions they advocate come from the most robust level of evidence examined objectively and critically before being put into healthcare practice. By using a care bundle, nurses may be confident that they are implementing the most relevant and effective care for their patients. In veterinary nursing, not only may it be difficult to access evidence-based practice, but due to the immature state of the profession, the evidence may simply not exist. It is for this reason that care bundles may be aspirational at this stage in veterinary nursing. There are several care bundles used widely in human-centred medicine that may, in time, be relevant to veterinary practice once the relevant evidence can be sourced. They include bundles for central venous catheter care, urinary catheter care, prevention of surgical site infection, and treatment of sepsis.

In 2013, Sarah Hancill [6] investigated the use of a care bundle for peripheral intravenous catheter patient safety in veterinary patients. Peripheral venous catheters (PVCs) are widely used in veterinary practice to gain intravenous access. There is established evidence in human-centred practice that there are associated risks of using PVC's, complications may lead to infection both locally and systemically. It is only logical that such findings may be extrapolated to apply to veterinary practice as well. In fact, complications may be more likely in animals as they are unable to be instructed to self-care for cannula sites and may indeed be their own source of infection should they lick or chew at the cannula site. In medical practice, the use of care bundles has reduced the incidence of PVC-associated infections. Again, it is only natural to surmise that application of a similar bundle may have the same beneficial effect in veterinary patients. The research presented by Hancill demonstrated that the use of a care bundle resulted in better care through an increase in quality indicators such as an increase in checking the catheter insertion site. Her conclusions centred on the challenges of implementation of the new tool for practice, rather than establishing if applying care bundles actually improved patient outcomes. She established that there was a relatively poor uptake of the care bundles in practice. She concluded that the main barrier for the use of care bundles was, in fact, staff behaviour. Her research demonstrates the importance of implementing change slowly and carefully, ensuring that all stakeholders are aware of why they are being asked to use the tool and the potential benefits the tool may provide for patient care. There is clearly scope for assessing if such a care bundle, implemented with due care and attention, may have an impact on clinical outcomes.

Integrated care pathways (ICP)

Integrated care pathways are another tool used regularly in human-centred healthcare that may have an application in veterinary medicine. Originally designed to facilitate the work of the multidisciplinary team, care pathways were first used in the mid 1980s in America and, since 1992, have been used throughout the NHS in a variety of clinical settings. Walsh [7] explains that in developing a care pathway all the professional groups involved in patient care are bought together and arrive at consensus about standards of care and specific evidence-based outcomes in selected patient groups within an agreed timeframe. They were introduced as a means of assisting healthcare professionals to deliver high quality, evidence-based, cost-effective care [8].

A care pathway is a document that stays with a patient throughout their care, as opposed to a care bundle which is implemented for a specific care need. It negates the need for individual standardised care plans for each nursing intervention, as all anticipated care needs are contained within the one document. Consider a patient admitted to a surgical ward from intensive care after cardiothoracic surgery. Such a patient is likely to require strict measurement of their fluid balance, intra venous medication, management of chest drains, and management of intra-nasal oxygen, all combined with ongoing support with more basic care needs such as personal care, eating, and drinking. If a standardised care plan is instigated for each of these interventions the pile of paperwork is set to be enormous. A care pathway provides an edited version of such care plans, edited with the needs of a specific group of patients in mind.

ICPs promote multidisciplinary working. This is in direct contrast to a nursing care plan which is exclusively aimed at nursing care, neglecting the input of other team members.

An integrated care pathway relies on the multidisciplinary team members keeping it updated. Without contemporary record keeping, there is a real danger of substandard care, omission of care, or perhaps, more dangerously, duplication of care.

An example of an integrated care pathway is the care that may be implemented should a patient suffer a heart attack and attend a hospital for primary percutaneous coronary intervention (PPCI). Figure 10.3 provides just a selection of pages from a PPCI integrated care pathway document to illustrate the variety of different elements of care that are covered. Additional sheets not demonstrated here include an observations chart for during the procedure, additional communications sheets, and post procedure care sheets immediately after the procedure, then for day zero, one, two and three.

PPCI involves the use of angiography to examine and potentially treat blockages in vessels in the heart, restoring blood flow. This is a time-dependent intervention, left too long without effective blood supply the heart is in danger of incurring permanent ischemic damage that may leave a patient in heart failure which will have significant effects on their quality and longevity of life. ICPs coordinate the application of evidence-based interventions from members of the multidisciplinary team, supporting a swift, collaborative intervention. The interventions are evidence-based and the team have clear guidance on what to do and when. A holistic approach is encouraged as the pathway leads the patient through from their acute admission with a handover from paramedic crew directly to the interventional radiographers, to the nursing staff who support patient recovery, to the interventions on health promotion from cardiac rehabilitation staff the day after their heart attack. Finally, the ICP incorporates planning of care once the patient has been discharged from the hospital and recovered from their acute illness, by including records of referrals made to the general practitioner for support in weight loss, diabetes management or smoking cessation.

Such tools may be useful in veterinary practice, particularly in a referral practice, where elective surgical interventions are planned ahead and may result in patients receiving a similar pathway of care. Orthopaedic cases lend themselves to the development of an ICP. All elements of the care should be taken into account, from admission to diagnostics, which may include imaging, or preanaesthetic screening, preparation for the procedure such as pre-medication and intravenous access, to induction of anaesthesia, maintenance of anaesthesia, and post-operative recovery. The next stage in the process may include wound management, post-operative imaging, referral to physiotherapy or hydrotherapy, and finally, education of owners for post-operative exercise and management at home. Nonclinical interventions may also be incorporated such as a financial planning section where conversations surrounding estimates and payment plans may be recorded.

The key point about integrated care pathways is their ability to facilitate a holistic and multidisciplinary approach to the patient, by inclusion of MDT input. Therefore, it is essential when writing such a care pathway, that all stakeholders are involved: nurses, vets, surgeons, anaesthetists, nursing assistants, physiotherapists and, if possible, owners of animals. Only then is the pathway likely to provide a true representation of the care the patient requires.

Patient Name:	Papworth Hospital **NHS**
Date of Birth:	NHS Foundation Trust
Hospital No:	
NHS No:	

Integrated Care Pathway
Primary Percutaneous Coronary Intervention (PPCI)

On arrival:

| Symptoms suggestive of STEMI? | Y / N |
| ECG consistent with STEMI / LBBB | Y / N |

Paramedic transfer:

Heparin 5000 Units:	Y / N
Aspirin 300mg:	Y / N
Clopidogrel 600 mg	Y / N
IV Access	Y / N
IV Opiates given:	Y / N
Fentanyl ....microgram	given at ....
Vomited	Y / N
Rhythm Problems	Y / N

Past Medical History

MI:	Y / N
Previous Coronary Angiogram	Y / N
PCI	Y / N
CABG:	Y / N
Diabetes:	Y / N
Hypertension:	Y / N
Renal problems:	Y / N
GI bleed or ulcers	Y / N
Intracranial pathology e.g. tumour / stroke	Y / N
Elective surgery planned	Y / N

Abbreviated Clinical Examination:

Alert & orientated?	Y / N
Airway safe?	Y / N
Pulse >50 and bilaterally symmetrical?	Y / N
SBP >100mmHg	Y / N
Signs of pulmonary congestion?	Y / N
Murmur?	Y / N

Consent:

| Verbal   /   Written |

Signature .... Date .... Time ....

ND131 PPCI ICP V5
File Section: 2
Updated on: 20th December 2012

Page 1 of 25

Figure 10.3 Papworth percutaneous primary coronary intervention care bundle. (Reproduced from Papworth Hospital NHS Foundation Trust. With kind permission.)

(Continued)

Patient Name:	Papworth Hospital **NHS**
Date of Birth:	NHS Foundation Trust
Hospital No:	
NHS No:	

Post PCI Procedure Guidelines	Date, Time & Sign
Attach to cardiac monitor ECG on return to ward and if further chest pain Base line observations – then half hourly for at least 2 hours Check sheath site Give clear fluids to drink – at least 1 litre over 4 hours Offer patient food 1 hour after return from procedure – time .... Pressure areas assessed Hygiene needs met Ensure patients and their families are kept informed and reassurance given If Primary PCI patient must not mobilise for 12 hours – time	
Femoral Sheath in Situ	
Patient to lie flat ACT 4 hours post last dose of Heparin ACT Time .... Result................ Repeat in 1 hr........... Result.............. If below 175 sheath can be removed. If above 175 repeat every 30 minutes until below 175. Give Atropine 600 mcgs IV (if prescribed) prior to sheath removal if heart rate below 60 bpm (if not administered keep by patients bedside) Sheath removed: Time .... By............ Half hourly observations for at least 2 hours Lie flat for 1 hour post sheath removal Sit up after 1 hour and offer food and drink Mobilise after 1 hour if haemostasis achieved or 12 hours if post MI Mobilise after a further 1 hour if haemostasis achieved or 12 hours if post MI Teach patient to self monitor puncture site	
Angioseal	
Patient to lie flat 30 minutes post deployment Patient to mobilise after 3 to 4 hours bed rest if haemostasis achieved or 12 hours if post MI Patient to be given angioseal advice card	
Radial	
Patient can sit in chair if they wish or bed rest for 12 hours if post MI Support affected arm with pillows If TR band in situ: **DIAGNOSTICS:** • Leave for 1 hour then remove 2 mls of air. • After 2 hours remove remaining air slowly over 1 minute. • Leave for 5 minutes then remove device by inflating band with 15 mls of air and then gently rolling it off. • If it bleeds, reinflate with sufficient air to stop bleeding. **PCI:** • Leave for 2 hours then remove 2 mls of air. • After a further hour remove 1-2 mls of air. • After a further half hour remove remaining air slowly over 1 minute. • Leave for 5 minutes then remove device by inflating band with 15 mls of air and then gently rolling it off.	

Figure 10.3 (*Continued*) Papworth percutaneous primary coronary intervention care bundle. (Reproduced from Papworth Hospital NHS Foundation Trust. With kind permission.)

Patient Name:	Papworth Hospital **NHS**
Date of Birth:	NHS Foundation Trust
Hospital No:	
NHS No:	

Date/Time	Communication Sheet (Information given to patient and relatives, critical incidents or accidents)	Signature and Designation

Figure 10.3 (*Continued*) Papworth percutaneous primary coronary intervention care bundle. (Reproduced from Papworth Hospital NHS Foundation Trust. With kind permission.)

(Continued)

Patient Name:

Date of Birth:

Hospital No:

NHS No:

Papworth Hospital **NHS**
NHS Foundation Trust

POST PROCEDURE: DAY 1 Date:	AM		PM		Nocte	
	Time	Initials	Time	Initials	Time	Initials
Cardiac monitor for at least 12 hours post procedure. Continue if patient condition warrants.						
Encourage patient to inform staff if they have any pain.						
Record ECG and repeat if any chest pain.						
Record observations as per cardiology guidelines or as patient warrants.						
Record patients actual weight:_____						
Fluid intake and output to be recorded Y / N						
Examine puncture / site. Refer to doctor if: • wound still oozing ++ • haematoma/swelling • lack of adjacent pulse						
Pressure areas assessed (if braden score < 12 start care plan)						
Hygiene needs met.						
Ensure patient and their families are kept informed and reassurance given at all times.						
Day 1 cardiac rehabilitation information given. Ensure patient has seen the BHF 'Life after a Heart Attack' DVD. (Give targeted health information sheet with relevant BHF books).						
Discuss discharge arrangements						
Bloods taken if applicable.						
Complete administration of ReoPro (Abciximab) / Angiox (Bivalirudin) checklist.						
Check cannula site & record VIP score						
Echo done: Yes / No / Requested (please circle) Ejection %						

Nurse signature AM	Nurses signature PM	Nurses signature Nocte
Print Name	Print Name	Print Name

Figure 10.3 (Continued) **Papworth percutaneous primary coronary intervention care bundle. (Reproduced from Papworth Hospital NHS Foundation Trust. With kind permission.)**

Patient Name:	Papworth Hospital **NHS**
Date of Birth:	NHS Foundation Trust
Hospital No:	
NHS No:	

POST PROCEDURE: DAY 3 Date:	AM		PM		Nocte	
	Time	Initials	Time	Initials	Time	Initials
Cardiac monitor for at least 12 hours. Continue if patient condition warrants.						
Encourage patient to inform staff if they have any pain.						
Record ECG and repeat if any chest pain.						
Record observations as per cardiology guidelines or as patient warrants.						
Examine puncture / site. Refer to doctor if: • wound still oozing ++ • haematoma/swelling • lack of adjacent pulse						
Pressure areas assessed (if Braden score < 12 start care plan)						
Hygiene needs met.						
Stair assessment done						
Ensure patient has seen the BHF 'Life after a Heart Attack' DVD.						
Ensure Phase One Cardiac Rehab given Yes / No						
Ensure patient and their families are kept informed and reassurance given at all times.						
Bloods taken if applicable.						
Check cannula site and record VIP score						
Comments						

Nurse signature AM	Nurses signature PM	Nurses signature Nocte
Print Name	Print Name	Print Name

Figure 10.3 (*Continued*) **Papworth percutaneous primary coronary intervention care bundle. (Reproduced from** Papworth Hospital NHS Foundation Trust. With kind permission.)

(*Continued*)

<table>
<tr><td colspan="2">Patient Name:

Date of Birth:

Hospital No:

NHS No:</td><td colspan="2" align="right">Papworth Hospital **NHS**
NHS Foundation Trust</td></tr>
</table>

	Cardiac Rehabilitation	Date & sign
	Phase 1 information discussed	
	Rehab centre referred to	

Targeted Health Education

Risk factor	Guidelines and advice given	
Post procedure blood pressure: _____ Ideal below140/85 mmHg (If diabetic, see below.)	BHF leaflet on Blood Pressure	☐
	You have been started on a drug to help reduce your blood pressure OR your current blood pressure medication has been altered.	☐
	You have been started on a drug to help to protect your heart which can also lower your blood pressure.	☐
	Please ask your Practice Nurse to check your blood pressure in a week's time and then as advised.	☐
	Blood pressure medication:	
Your total cholesterol: _____ Ideal below 5.0mmol/l	BHF leaflet on Reducing your Blood Cholesterol	☐
Your LDL cholesterol: _____ Ideal below 3.0mmol/l	You have been started on a cholesterol lowering tablet.	☐
	You have had your cholesterol lowering medication increased or altered.	☐
	Please make an appointment with your GP or Practice Nurse to have your cholesterol levels checked in 12 weeks time.	☐
	To further reduce your cholesterol levels you are advised to maintain a low fat diet. Cholesterol medication: _____	
Your weight: _____Kg	BHF leaflet on Eating for your Heart	☐
Your body mass index: _____ Ideal between 20-25	We advise you to lose weight. Please see your GP, Practice Nurse or Cardiac Rehabilitation team who can help you with this. Your ideal weight should be between: _____ Kg	☐
Diabetes Diabetes type I / type II Ideal BP below 130/80	BHF booklet on Diabetes and your Heart Your diabetes treatment: _____	☐
HbA1C result:	Referral to Community Diabetic Nurse required Yes / No	☐
Current smoker: Yes / No	BHF leaflet Smoking and your Heart	☐
Smoking amount: _____ Smoking duration: _____	Please see your Practice Nurse or Cardiac Rehabilitation team for help to stop smoking. Camquit Telephone number: **0800 018 4304**	☐
Stopped when? _____	Referral to Smoking Cessation is required Yes / No	☐
Other risks Stress / Exercise Alcohol	Stress Management leaflet given BHF booklet Physical activity and your Heart Your average weekly intake in units has been: _____	☐ ☐

Please tick: Tomcat version completed   Paper Version ICP completed

Figure 10.3 (Continued) **Papworth percutaneous primary coronary intervention care bundle. (Reproduced from Papworth Hospital NHS Foundation Trust. With kind permission.)**

Patient Name:				
Date of Birth:				
Hospital No:			Papworth Hospital NHS	
NHS No:			NHS Foundation Trust	

Discharge

Expected day of discharge ....

Actual day of discharge ....

Time of discharge ....

Discharged on PAS: ....

		Date & time	Initials
Clinical Assessment	Cannula removed Yes / No		
	Examine groin / Radial site (if any concerns Dr to review before discharge) Yes / No		
	Advice for site care given Yes / No		
	Give Angioseal card Yes / No / NA		
Medication	TTO's: Yes / No Given / Not Given		
	Discharge medication checked and explained (inclu. GTN spray)? Yes / No		
	Explain importance & reason for taking Clopidogrel post PCI. Yes / No		
	Give Clopridogrel card. Yes / No		
	Metformin to commence 48 hours post procedure Date		
	Warfarin to recommence on:...............		
	Daily dosage to be written on TTO's until next INR appointment (If patient new to Warfarin, ensure they have had counselling via Pharmacist)		
	Warfarin appt. Date .... Time .... Place		
	Patient Warfarin book completed Yes / No		
Discharge Plan	Referred to Cardiac Rehab Yes / No		
	Patient for outpatient surgery? Yes / No If yes, cardiac support referral completed? Yes / No		
	Transport Booked Date .... Time		
	Discharge feedback obtained Yes / No		
Safety	If MI advised no driving for 4 weeks from date of MI Yes / No / NA		
	If PCI advised no driving for 1 week from date of procedure Yes / No / NA		
	Health promotion advice given Yes / No		
	Stairs assessment done Yes / No		
Nurse Signature		Print Name	
Date		Time	

Figure 10.3 (Continued) Papworth percutaneous primary coronary intervention care bundle. (Reproduced from Papworth Hospital NHS Foundation Trust. With kind permission.)

Concept mapping

Concept maps are diagrams that represent, produce, and organise knowledge. They are visual aids to link information together to be able to demonstrate an overview of a situation. It has been proposed that concept mapping may be a useful framework to structure care planning and case conferencing. Care management is becoming increasingly complex due to a number of factors, such as, the advancing average age of patients. This means many people now have multiple co-morbidities and the increased health promotion services provided by the healthcare systems results in a greater number of professionals having an input into care planning.

Concept mapping puts the patient at the centre of care planning, both virtually and literally, on the diagram. Such representation is done to encourage a patient-centred approach so that the patient's perspective is always considered in relation to what they perceive their problem to be and how it affects them. This is important as the perception of the health-related problem of the patient may indeed be different to that of the healthcare team. It is a tool that may be used after comprehensive assessment to analyse information gathered, identify and include any extra information, and identify any deficits in information.

The format of concept mapping involves consideration of how a person's life story, health, environment and social wellbeing may combine to enable or disable them. It encourages the team to work with the patient using their strengths to improve their situation.

Concept mapping may provide a documented record of clinical decision making, providing evidence should nursing decisions be challenged at a later date. The process of concept mapping relies upon a knowledgeable facilitator conversant with the process. That facilitator must gather both information about the patient and the relevant staff members to map the patients' needs and plan how they will be addressed. The emphasis will be on using facts, challenging assumptions, and ensuring the care plan remains patient-centred. The facilitator will also be responsible for ensuring that clear outcomes are developed and taken forward. Care plans must be adjusted immediately and follow up actions agreed for the process to have any credibility.

A marked criticism of concept mapping is the aesthetics of the resulting diagram (Figure 10.4). They are generally busy and complicated and the appearance may prevent staff members who were not involved with the process from using the tool. Staff may prefer to compartmentalise and categorise the different care needs of the patient, however, care must be taken not to lose the joined-up approach the concept map is trying to promote.

Clinical applications of concept mapping may be limited in veterinary nursing, where multidisciplinary case conferences about specific patients are rare. They may be useful within a different context of veterinary care: emergency care planning, in particular when team members are not used to working with each other. The use of locum staff may be a barrier to cohesive teamworking as members of the team may have never met each other before and yet need to work in an intense environment with critically ill patients. Once stabilised, a concept map of the care a patient needs may be a swift way of assigning tasks to team members and ensuring that all care needs are met.

There is certainly an argument to use concept maps in veterinary nurse education. They are a clear demonstration of how holistic care may support a patient's return to health. The process stimulates the recognition of connections between care needs and care interventions. It may help students to develop a thought process whereby actual and potential problems are linked to the patients' health, environment and general life story.

Concept mapping may be an excellent leadership tool for a practice team to begin to develop new ideas and strategies. With key values or objectives at the centre of the concept map, a multidisciplinary, joined-up approach to achieving a new way of working may be developed.

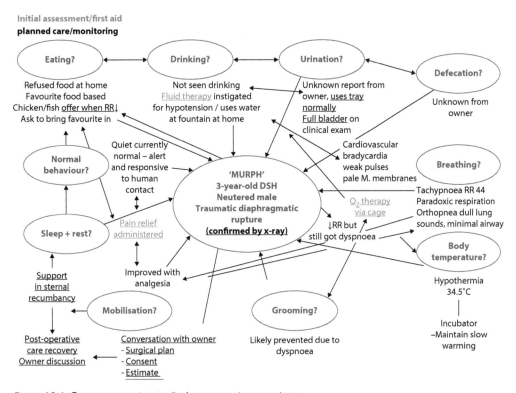

Figure 10.4 Concept mapping applied to a veterinary patient.

Is the nursing care plan redundant?

In the interest of critical thinking, the question that should be asked is, should integrated care bundles and care pathways replace nursing care plans? The answer is overwhelmingly, no. They must be used in conjunction with, and as an adjuvant to, nursing care plans and the care planning process. A care bundle is linked to a very specific intervention or set of symptoms that a patient is experiencing. To implement a care bundle in a patient without a comprehensive assessment could lead to omissions in care and neglect of primitive care needs. Equally, integrated care pathways should always incorporate an element of nursing assessment to ensure that patient health and welfare is supported. Concept maps are a different form of planning care and may be used in conjunction with a nursing model so that the veterinary team may be sure that they are providing holistic care.

In practice

Didzy is a 12-year-old Jack Russel Terrier who has been admitted for an elective cruciate repair. This is exactly the type of procedure that may utilise an integrated care pathway, as each member of the team may play a role in the patient's care. Initially, the nurse admits the patient and, using the Ability Model, makes a note of certain individual traits that Didzy has. In particular, the nurse makes a note of the fact that he will only eat dry food and is almost completely deaf. Furthermore, the owner describes how Didzy can sometimes become fearful should he be surprised and may bite.

Imagine the consequences should this information not be collected and subsequently passed on to the team caring for Didzy, a scenario real enough if the cruciate ICP had simply been instigated without a nursing assessment. Staff may have been at risk from Didzy because if they didn't realise he was deaf, they may have surprised him by appearing at his kennel when he hadn't heard them. Offering him tinned food after his anaesthesia would have meant a hungry dog, given that he only eats dry food. While each of these points may not be life threatening, they affect the health and wellbeing of both the patient and the veterinary staff.

Individualised care

An important objection to care bundles and integrated care pathways, reported anecdotally, is their uniform nature. They are designed to take advantage of common characteristics of one condition or set of symptoms (Figure 10.5). Implementing a care bundle or integrated care pathway allows staff to take advantage of recurrent patterns within healthcare to support patients who need similar interventions. They shouldn't replace an initial conversation either with the patient or with the patient's owner to understand the unique needs of that patient. Not all patients require the same treatment and therefore a care bundle, like all treatments, requires careful critical thinking to ensure that nurses understand the treatment they are giving as well as the implications of the care. Assumptions about the care needs of a patient based on their diagnosis shouldn't be made. Care planning requires high quality assessment to implement individualised, relevant and effective interventions. Some of those interventions may well be the implementation of a specific care pathway or care bundles, but without that initial assessment, how would a nurse know which care bundles to apply? One particular example is the policy of the administration of deep veined thrombosis prophylaxis treatment to patients admitted to hospital in the UK. According to the NICE guideline [9] patients should be assessed for their risk of developing an embolism and preventative treatment given appropriately. This can quickly become routine practice for a large majority of patients on a ward. It can be easy to assume that all patients will need such preventative treatment. However, some patients should not be given such treatment, if their condition is linked to bleeding or they are bleeding after a procedure, and while this seems obvious, it does require attention to the individual situation of the patient as it is easy to default to the prevention treatment.

Interestingly, to take account of this need for a truly holistic assessment, one of the key recommendations of a chronic obstructive pulmonary disease (COPD) care bundle is a referral to the specialist respiratory nurse. These nurses will perform a holistic and comprehensive assessment to facilitate the best care to try and prevent future exacerbations of COPD. They will ascertain whether a patient needs oxygen at home, find out if they are still smoking, establish if they need help with their activities of living, such as preparing meals to eat, washing and dressing. While appetite is not on the care bundle, it is an essential part of preventing exacerbation. Malnutrition may lead to an immunocompromised patient which may leave them vulnerable to infection, and chest infections are cause of exacerbations of COPD. A care bundle will not take that into account. However, a nursing model of care, designed to support patients with chronic respiratory disease in the community will facilitate a holistic approach through use of the nursing process.

Nursing care plan	Concept mapping	Care bundles	Integrated care pathways
Use a nursing model to assess the whole patient	Uses a nursing model to assess the whole patient	Used for a specific patient group, disease or set of symptoms	Useful for complex care that follows a set pattern requiring multi-disciplinary input
Individualised care	Individualised care	Standardised care for a patient group	Standardised care for a patient group
Not always evidence based	Not always evidence based	Always evidence based	Always evidence based
Freehand descriptive record of care, allowing for subjective observations	Freehand descriptive record of care, allowing for subjective observations	Checklist style record of care	Checklist style record of care
Not always useful for clinical audit	Complicated presentation of data may make it difficult to use for clinical audit	Usually useful for clinical audit	Usually useful for clinical audit

Figure 10.5 **Characteristics of nursing care plans, concept mapping, care bundles and integrated care pathways.**

Actual and potential problems

The key point is that the nursing staff must be able to recognise the needs of a patient. Care planning is anticipatory and proactive, allowing the nursing team to develop strategies for both actual and potential problems. They need to be able to think critically and analyse the information they have received about a patient. Each of these skills is facilitated through the use of nursing models in planning care. Models such as RLT and, in veterinary nursing, the Ability Model, encourage nurses to take into account extra influencing factors such as psychological care, financial situation, compliance and social factors. It is these factors that individualise care and make it relevant and more effective for a patient.

Narrative skills

Equally important is maintaining the narrative skills of nurse record keeping. While care bundles and care pathways may minimise the need for descriptive writing, documentation of communication with the patient, their family and friends is essential to maintain a continuity of care and ensure all relevant information is shared appropriately. Therefore it is important that nurses do not lose their narrative writing skills.

The future of care planning – Using information technology

Alongside the use of new tools to support care planning, such as the care bundle and ICP, new technologies are being used to support different methods of care planning.

Electronic whiteboards

Electronic or interactive whiteboards are large electronic wall-mounted displays that provide patient-specific information to healthcare staff. Dry wipe boards are often used on hospital wards to provide details of patients, however, they have been criticised as labour-intensive, out of date, and unreliable as data, once erased from the board, is lost forever. Electronic white boards have been used in healthcare to provide real-time information about the status of both individual patients and entire departments or hospitals. This enables the healthcare staff to plan care on a wider, departmental level and can allow for direct prioritisation of care needs amongst groups of patients.

They are complex tools that, like nursing care plans, must be introduced carefully to ensure that they become useful tools, rather than a hindrance or source of stress. Departments must decide what information should be recorded, whether it will be manually or automatically updated, and in what format the information is displayed. Potentially, combining a nursing care plan onto such a tool will combat one of the biggest barriers to the use of nursing care plans, the fact that they quickly become out of date. Nurses will be able to update care plans as they change.

Electronic whiteboards have the advantage being able to improve patient safety through the effective dissemination of patient information, which insures that the care needs of patients are not missed. They can reduce the need for constant internal updates amongst staff, freeing them up for patient care, as information is contemporary and quickly available. They promote the principles of patient confidentiality, as security measures can be put in place to ensure that exposure to members of the public is minimal.

Collaborative interactive technology

The development of specialist centres for human-centred health in the UK has necessitated the need for hospitals to develop tools that allow medical teams to obtain advice and guidance in planning care for certain patient groups. As an example, the author has witnessed the use of video conferencing to allow a specialist burns team from a specialist trauma centre 30 miles away from a general hospital to assess a patient and guide the local team to implement a care plan of elective intubation before transferring the patient to a specialist burns unit.

Information technology can be used to share imaging, CT scans, MRI scans, and x-rays so that real-time assessment of diagnostic test results can be carried out by multiple members of the patient's medical team at different sites. Such tools facilitate true multidisciplinary team care planning, both with the team caring for the patient at the time as well as involvement of extra team members who may be consulted for bespoke specialist advice. Nurses may request the input of specialist services, such as a psychiatrist or social worker, based on their initial assessment, and individualised patient-centred care can be planned with the experts, all in one go. Such care planning must surely facilitate a smoother care pathway for the patient as any internal conflict may be addressed at the time. So, while a psychiatrist may be keen to see a patient as they have expressed suicidal thoughts, a consultant may have only one slot in which to facilitate a specific diagnostic test. Being able to talk that through in real time allows priorities to be set and patient needs addressed according to both the health status of the individual and, most importantly, their expressed needs.

The expert patient

One final tool, well-used by the NHS but currently neglected within veterinary practice, is the use of the patient. Throughout human-centred healthcare, more and more patients are being welcomed into medical teams to provide their unique input as services are evaluated and modified. Patients are key stakeholders in the services that provide them with their care. Patient support groups provide a supportive environment where people suffering from similar conditions may share experiences and exchange information and advice. Increasingly, medical professionals are realising that they may learn from their patients and develop their practice accordingly.

In planning a package of care to be implemented for patients who are being discharged from surgery, it is useful to ascertain which services have been most useful for promoting rehabilitation. When designing a new chronic health care plan, surely one of the most important groups of stakeholders to consult is the patients? The patients will be using the care plans and therefore it is natural that patients have an input into what is included in the plan.

The same applies to veterinary nursing. Nursing chronically ill patients requires careful care planning. Consultation with the owners of such patients can provide a useful insight into the types of services the practice can provide that would help them care for their animal, the use of a home care plan for example. Some owners struggle to remember when to give medication, so development of a home medication chart might be useful to help owners plan the administration of their pet's medication. Might it be worth having a diabetic-themed meeting, or a mini conference on the care of patients with chronic renal failure where owners of patients experiencing these problems may come together and exchange experiences? From the experiences of the NHS, such meetings may provide both support and comfort for patient owners, but also key strategies and ideas for the veterinary team to implement to provide a more robust patient-centred service.

There are many tools available with the aim of optimising the use of resources and supporting the delivery of effective patient care. One thing remains essential to the healthcare of people or animals, the ability to think, to process, and weigh up information. Nursing is an art based on science and the art surely must be that initial assessment. The process of looking at a patient and planning the care they need requires a combination of knowledge, experience, intuition and science. Diagnostic tests support the process and provide the science through demonstration of the physiological needs of the patient, but only assessment of the patient will inform the nurse whether in fact a physiological deficit is actually affecting their patient's quality of life. Nursing requires both art and science; holistic care cannot be achieved without them.

Review

- Contemporary care planning tools have been developed to account for increased multidisciplinary input for patients who have complex care needs.
- Care bundles and integrated care pathways use evidence-based medicine to guide clinical interventions, however, they must be used in conjunction with the individualised care needs each unique patient has.
- The use of care bundles and integrated care pathways may improve clinical outcomes, but also can have nonclinical benefits for the healthcare team.
- Concept mapping is a valuable educational tool for demonstrating a holistic and multidisciplinary approach to nursing care.
- Information technology provides valuable resources for sharing skills across different working environments so that specialist review and opinion may be sought early into the care planning process.

Further reflections

Is there a particular clinical intervention in practice that is often subject to debate and discussion? Do some nurses use different methods and achieve different results? Consider the different resources they use for this intervention, the different knowledge they have, and where and how they learned their knowledge. Perform a review of the literature or evidence available surrounding the intervention. There may be a range of different resources available to gather evidence depending on the intervention. If related to a particular product or piece of equipment, consider approaching the company representatives and asking whether they have any evidence to support their product. Enquire with your practice manager whether the practice has any subscriptions to online resources that you may be able to use to access nursing journals. Consider linking through to human-centred nursing studies on the same subject to establish whether there is any information that may be extrapolated and applied to animals. Examine the evidence critically, thinking about bias and quality to gather robust evidence surrounding the intervention. Discuss your findings with the rest of the nursing team and see whether a consensus may be reached and then formalised by the use of a care bundle.

References

1. Norman B (2010). An Ounce of Prevention: Best Practice Bundles. Retrieved from https://www .amsn.org/sites/default/files/private/medsurg-matters-newsletter-archives/marapr10.pdf.
2. Institute of Healthcare Improvement (2012). How to Guide: Prevent Ventilator Associated Pneumonia. Retrieved from http://www.ihi.org/resources/pages/tools/howtoguidepreventvap .aspx.
3. Clarkson D (2013). The role of 'care bundles' in healthcare. *British Journal of Healthcare Management*, 19, 63–68.
4. Dellinger RP et al. (2013). Surviving sepsis campaign: International guidelines for management of severer sepsis and septic shock: 2012. *Critical Care Medicine*, 41, 580–637.
5. Levy MM et al. (2010). The surviving sepsis campaign: Results of an international guideline-based performance improvement program targeting severe sepsis. *Intensive Care Medicine*, 36 (2), 222–231.
6. Hancill S (2013). Peripheral intravenous catheters: Improving patient safety with the use of a care bundle. *Veterinary Nurse*, 4 (7), 436–441.
7. Walsh M (1998). *Models and Critical Pathways in Clinical Nursing*. Edinburgh: Bailliere Tindall.
8. Kozier B et al. (2008). *Fundamentals of Nursing, Concepts, Processes and Practice*. Harlow: Pearson Education.
9. National Institute of Health and Care Excellence (2010). Venous Thromboembolism Reducing the Risk for Patients in Hospital [online]. Last accessed 29th March 2017. https://www.nice.org.uk/ Guidance/CG92.

Further reading

Learning from the experiences of human-centred nurses may help the veterinary nursing profession move forward effectively.

1. *Clinical Information Systems in Critical Care. Cecily Morrison, Matthew Jones, Julie Bracken (Cambridge University Press, 2014).*

Index

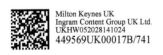